Management of the Acutely Ill Neurological Patient

Management of the Acutely Ill Neurological Patient

Edited by

James C. Grotta, M.D.
Professor
Department of Neurology
University of Texas Medical School at Houston
Director
Stroke Program
Hermann Hospital
Houston, Texas

Churchill Livingstone
New York, Edinburgh, London, Madrid, Melbourne, Tokyo

Library of Congress Cataloging-in-Publication Data

Management of the acutely ill neurological patient / edited by James
   C. Grotta.
      p.   cm.
   Includes bibiliographical references and index.
   ISBN 0-443-08870-5
   1. Neurological intensive care.   I. Grotta, James C.
   [DNLM: 1. Central Nervous System Diseases—therapy. 2. Acute
Disease—therapy. WL 300 M266 1993]
   RC350.N49M36   1993
   616.8'0428—dc20
   DNLM/DLC
   for Library of Congress   93-9652
                                           CIP

Distributed in the United Kingdom by Churchill Livingstone, Robert Stevenson
House, 1–3 Baxter's Place, Leith Walk, Edinburgh EH1 3AF, and by associated compa-
nies, branches, and representatives throughout the world.

Accurate indications, adverse reactions, and dosage schedules for drugs are provided
in this book, but it is possible that they may change. The reader is urged to review the
package information data of the manufacturers of the medications mentioned.

The Publishers have made every effort to trace the copyright holders for borrowed
material. If they have inadvertently overlooked any, they will be pleased to make the
necessary arrangements at the first opportunity.

Acquisitions Editor: *Nancy Mullins*
Copy Editor: *Barbara L. B. Storey and Lorene K. Johnson*
Production Supervisor: *Patricia McFadden*
Cover Design: *Paul Moran*

Printed in the United States of America

First published in 1993   7   6   5   4   3   2   1

To Kathy, Amy, Jacob, and Andrew, with apologies for all the times I've missed dinner; and to our "stroke team" (Patti, Linda, Bill, Creed, Dan, Carmela, Tom, Sandy, Mark, and Frank), who have helped redefine acute neurological care.

Contributors

Karen M. Andrews, M.D.
Fellow in EMG and Neuromuscular Disease, Department of Neurology, University of Texas Medical School at Houston, Houston, Texas

Sara G. Austin, M.D.
Assistant Professor, Department of Neurology, University of Texas Medical School at Houston; Chief, Department of Neurology, Lyndon Baines Johnson General Hospital, Houston, Texas

David S. Baskin, M.D., F.A.C.S.
Associate Professor, Departments of Neurology and Anesthesiology, Baylor College of Medicine, Houston, Texas

Joseph Berger, M.D.
Professor, Departments of Neurology and Internal Medicine, University of Miami School of Medicine, Miami, Florida

James L. Bernat, M.D.
Professor, Department of Neurology, Dartmouth Medical School, Hanover, New Hampshire; Chief, Neurology Section, Veterans Administration Medical Center, White River Junction, Vermont

Jeffrey L. Clothier, M.D.
Assistant Professor, Department of Psychiatry, University of Arkansas College of Medicine, Little Rock, Arkansas

Michael P. Earnest, M.D.
Professor, Departments of Neurology and Preventive Medicine, University of Colorado School of Medicine; Director, Department of Neurology, Denver General Hospital, Denver, Colorado

James C. Grotta, M.D.
Professor, Department of Neurology, University of Texas Medical School at Houston; Director, Stroke Program, Hermann Hospital, Houston, Texas

Daniel F. Hanley, M.D.
Associate Professor, Departments of Neurology and Anesthesiology/Critical Care Medicine, Division of Neurosciences Critical Care, Johns Hopkins University School of Medicine; Director, Neurosciences Critical Care Unit, Department of Neurology, Johns Hopkins Hospital, Baltimore, Maryland

Sandra K. Hanson, M.D.
Cerebrovascular Fellow, Department of Neurology, University of Texas Medical School at Houston, Houston, Texas

Hilton R. Lacy, M.D.
Fellow, Department of Child Psychiatry, University of Virginia School of Medicine, Charlottesville, Virginia

Robert M. Levy, M.D., Ph.D.
Associate Professor, Departments of Neurosurgery and Physiology, Northwestern University Medical School, Chicago, Illinois

Russ P. Nockels, M.D.
Assistant Professor, Department of Neurological Surgery, University of California, San Francisco, School of Medicine, San Francisco, California

William D. Parker, Jr.,M.D.
Associate Professor, Department of Neurology, University of Colorado School of Medicine; Staff Pediatric Neurologist, Children's Hospital, Denver, Colorado

Lawrence H. Pitts, M.D.
Vice Chairman and Professor, Department of Neurological Surgery, University of California, San Francisco, School of Medicine, San Francisco, California

David M. Treiman, M.D.
Professor, Department of Neurology, University of California, Los Angeles, UCLA School of Medicine; Co-director, Veterans Affairs Southwest Regional Epilepsy Center, Veterans Affairs Medical Center, West Los Angeles, Los Angeles, California

Francine J. Vriesendorp, M.D.
Assistant Professor, Department of Neurology, University of Texas Medical School at Houston; Director, EMG Laboratory, Hermann Hospital, Houston, Texas

Michael A. Williams, M.D.
Instructor, Departments of Neurology and Anesthesiology/Critical Care Medicine, Division of Neurosciences Critical Care, Johns Hopkins University School of Medicine; Director, Clinical Neurocirculatory Laboratory, Department of Neurology, Johns Hopkins Hospital, Baltimore, Maryland

Preface

This book was conceived as a result of the dramatic changes now occurring in the practice of neurology. The development of rapid, precise, noninvasive diagnostic imaging, as well as reimbursement disincentives that discourage hospitalization strictly for diagnostic purposes, has changed neurological diagnosis into a largely ambulatory endeavor. Consequently, those patients who *are* admitted to the hospital with primary neurological illnesses tend to be more acutely ill than in the past.

The clinical care of patients hospitalized with acute neurological illnesses is also changing. Cost-containment methods favor rapid evaluation, treatment, and "discharge planning." More importantly, neurology is rapidly becoming a therapeutically oriented specialty in many cases because of increased ability to make rapid, precise diagnoses, improved understanding of the pathophysiology of acute neurological illnesses, and an expanding armamentarium of therapeutic options. While the neurological examination and accurate anatomic localization remain the foundations of neurological diagnosis, it is rare for teaching rounds to dwell primarily on these classical methods. Instead, discussion more often revolves around the results of MRI scans or transesophageal echocardiograms, ventilator settings or intracranial pressure management, or which platelet antiaggregant, anticonvulsant, or plasmapheresis regimen to choose.

The battleground of neurological care has shifted from the ward to the emergency room and intensive care unit. For some disorders, such as stroke, it may soon become the ambulance. The initial decisions about diagnostic evaluation and therapy are, in most cases, now made in the emergency room. Patients usually leave the emergency room with much of the diagnostic workup completed and therapy started. Neurological critical care units, either freestanding or part of larger medical or surgical critical care units, are now the initial destination of most acute neurological admissions. Consequently, neurologists commonly work side by side with emergency room physicians and intensivists, and all three groups need to speak the same language.

This book is written for emergency room physicians, intensivists, and all other non-neurologists who are called upon to help manage hospitalized patients with acute neurological illness. Hopefully, neurology students, residents, and staff will also find it useful for a "state-of-the-art" review. The chapters have been written by authorities in the specific fields, with instructions to address clinically relevant aspects of diagnosis, management, and treatment of adult and pediatric patients with acute neurological illness.

James C. Grotta, M.D.

Contents

1

Metabolic Encephalopathies and Coma from Medical Causes

Michael P. Earnest
William D. Parker, Jr.

[The brain] is specially the organ which enables us to think, see and hear. . . . It is the brain too which is the seat of madness and delirium, of the fears and frights which assail us, often by night, but sometimes even by day. . . . All such things result from an unhealthy condition of the brain.

Hippocrates of Cos
The Sacred Disease[1]

The brain is the organ that creates wakefulness, sleep, thought, memory, perception, insight, emotion, and behavior—in short, all the functions of the human mind. The brain's functions arise from the activity of approximately 100 billion complexly interconnected neurons supported by the glial cells, mainly astrocytes and myelin-producing oligodendrocytes. Neurons interact through electric impulses and chemical neurotransmitters. Both electric and chemical neurotransmission depend on a finely balanced intra- and extracellular milieu of electrolytes, water, hydrogen ions, amino acids, excitatory and inhibitory chemicals, and metabolic substrates. Proper physiologic function of neurons and glia also depends on maintenance of their milieu within a strict range of temperature, osmolality, pH, and blood flow. Any systemic metabolic derangement or intoxication can cause brain cellular dysfunction, and so cause disordered alertness, cognition, and behavior at the clinical level.[2]

Severe metabolic and toxic disorders lead to coma, irreversible brain injury, and in the extreme, brain death. Confused, delirious patients, compared with mentally intact ones, have longer hospital stays, are more likely to die, and more often are discharged to institutional care.[3, 4] A morbid outcome is especially common in the elderly.[3–5]

This chapter presents the clinical manifestations of metabolic encephalopathies in adults and children, their differential diagnosis, laboratory evaluation, and management. The evaluation, management, and prognosis of metabolically induced coma are all discussed separately because of the special clinical issues the comatose patient presents to the critical care physician.

CLINICAL DIAGNOSIS OF ENCEPHALOPATHY

Metabolic encephalopathies almost always begin clinically as delirium. *Delirium* is the currently preferred term, and is synonymous with *acute confusional state*. *Acute organic brain syndrome, acute brain disorder, clouded sensorium,* and many other commonly used terms should be dropped from the clinical vocabulary.

The cardinal feature of delirium is disordered cognitive function. The delirious patient usually also has impaired behavior, disturbed sleep–wake cycle, and in severe cases, sensory misperceptions and even hallucinations.[2, 6] Typically, the manifestations wax and wane throughout the day and are often worse at night. Physical signs include autonomic nervous system dysfunction and abnormal motor activity.[6]

Recognition of delirium relies on clinical observation. Delirium may be first suspected when the patient's behavior becomes disordered. The patient may attempt to pull out intravenous lines or endotracheal tubes or to get out of bed. Reversal or disruption of the sleep–wake cycle frequently occurs. The patient's conversation may become difficult to follow, and the patient may be less attentive and more distractable than normal.

If delirium is suspected, it should be confirmed by a careful mental status and neurological examination. The bedside mental status examination should include observations of the patient's level of alertness, psychomotor function, orientation, memory, attentiveness, thought patterns, and sensory perceptions. Alertness may be increased (e.g., the hypervigilant, hyperactive, delirium tremens patient) or decreased (e.g., the apathetic elderly patient). Orientation is tested for person, place, and time. Memory tests focus on ability to recall several items after 5 minutes (e.g., table, rose, 63 Broadway, and love) and memory of recent events (e.g., When were you admitted to the hospital? Who is your doctor? What did you have for dinner last night?).

Inattentiveness is often shown by the patient's incorrect responses to questions and instructions. Formal tests of attention include serial subtractions (i.e., serial 7's from 100 or 3's from 20), naming the months of the year backward, repeating four- and five-digit numbers in reverse, and spelling *world* backward. Thought pattern disorder is usually demonstrated by the patient's confused or rambling conversation and inappropriate responses to questions. Disordered perceptions may be cutaneous ("bugs on my skin"), visual ("spiders on the wall"), auditory (accusatory voices), or cognitive (e.g., misperceiving the physician or nurse as a family member).

Several formalized, brief, bedside mental status examinations have been developed.[7-9] These are probably no more sensitive than a thorough clinical examination. However, they nicely standardize the bedside evaluation of mental status, and can be administered by house staff, nurses, and students.

The assessment should also include the autonomic and motor signs of encephalopathy. Autonomic manifestations include fever, tachycardia, hypertension, tachypnea, and diaphoresis. Motor signs include tremor, asterixis, multifocal myoclonus, and seizures. Tremor and asterixis are best demonstrated by having the patient raise and extend the arms forward and dorsiflex the hands. Fine hand tremor or irregular lateral finger tremor is common. Asterixis occurs after at least 30 seconds of suspension, and is seen as a sudden, quick, downward jerk of the hands with a slower recovery to the dorsiflexed postion.[10] Multifocal myoclonus appears as irregular, quick, asynchronous, asymmetric jerks of the limbs and face, it is usually seen only in severe metabolic-toxic disorders. Convulsions are usually generalized (*grand mal*) and may be single or multiple. However, pre-existing focal brain lesions plus a superimposed encephalopathy may produce focal motor seizures. The remainder of the neurological examination, including cranial nerve, cerebellar strength, and sensory and tendon reflex testing, usually is not helpful. The appearance of bilateral Babinski signs is suggestive, but not diagnostic, of encephalopathy.

DIFFERENTIAL DIAGNOSIS AND LABORATORY EVALUATION

The patient with an encephalopathy causing delirium presents an extremely broad differential diagnosis. The most common causes are metabolic and toxic ones, but systemic and central nervous system (CNS) infections, structural brain lesions, psychiatric disorders, nonconvulsive or complex partial (temporal lobe) seizures, or unsuspected trauma may present with delirium as well.[2, 6] In recent years, patients with acquired immunodeficiency syndrome (AIDS) and delirium have presented new diagnostic challenges[11] (see Ch. 9). Table 1-1 lists the multiple etiologies that must be considered.

The initial steps in establishing a specific diagnosis include a complete medical history (e.g., prescribed medications and substance abuse history) and careful general medical neurological examinations. The general medical examination includes observation for signs of meningitis and other infections. The neurological examination, beyond the mental status examination, looks for papilledema and focal signs, such as hemiparesis, asymmetric reflexes, or a unilateral Babinski sign.

The laboratory work-up must be based on the specific clinical history and findings. In the typical patient with delirium of unknown cause, tests that should be performed are complete blood count, biochemical and electrolyte screens, blood and urine toxin screens, arterial blood gas, blood culture, a computed tomography (CT) scan of the head, and a lumbar puncture. More specific history or findings might indicate additional work-up (e.g., endocrine hormone levels, blood carboxyhemoglobin, human immunodeficiency virus [HIV] antibody titers, or specific drug blood levels [e.g., aspirin, alcohol, tricyclic drugs]). If a psychiatric disorder is suspected, an electroencephalogram (EEG) may be helpful. In most toxic-metabolic infections encephalopathy, the EEG shows diffuse slowing of the normal background rhythms, plus intermixed abnormal rhythms.[12] In psychiatric disease, the EEG is usually normal, in the absence of sedating or tranquilizing drugs.

Usually, a broad search for the etiology of delirium will disclose a specific, usually treatable etiology. However, in a significant minority of cases in an intensive care unit (ICU), no single or obvious cause is identified. The recommended clinical approach to that case is, once again, to thoroughly review the history and the patient's medical chart to ensure nothing has been overlooked, especially in the arena of substance abuse, exposure to unusual toxins, AIDS risk factors, or current medications that may be causing brain dysfunction. If still no etiology is found, a multifactorial encephalopathy must be considered (Table 1-1).

Table 1-1. COMMON METABOLIC, TOXIC, INFECTIOUS, NEUROLOGICAL, AND MISCELLANEOUS CAUSES OF DELIRIUM

I. Systemic Medical Disorders
  A. Metabolic substrate disorders
    1. Glucose—hypo- or hyperglycemia
    2. Hypoxia
  B. Electrolytes
    1. Sodium—hypo- or hypernatremia
    2. Calcium—hypo- or hypercalcemia
    3. Uncommonly hypermagnessemia or hypophosphatemia
  C. Acid–base balance
    1. Acidosis
    2. Alkalosis
  D. Specific organs
    1. Liver failure
    2. Uremia
    3. Lung failure (causing hypoxia, hypercarbia, acidosis)
    4. Rarely pancreatitis
  E. Endocrine systems
    1. Thyroid—hypo- or hyperactivity
    2. Adrenal insufficiency
    3. Pituitary failure
    4. Endocrine pancreas (causing hyperglycemia, acidosis)
  F. Autoimmune system
    1. Lupus erythematosus
    2. CNS vasculitis
  G. Blood flow and pressure
    1. Severe hypotension
    2. Severe anemia
    3. Hypertensive encephalopathy
    4. Cardiopulmonary bypass
  H. Miscellaneous
    1. Hyperosmolarity
    2. Severe hyper- or hypothermia
    3. Porphyria
    4. Fat emboli
    5. Noninfectious (marantic) endocarditis

(continued)

Table 1-1. COMMON METABOLIC, TOXIC, INFECTIOUS, NEUROLOGICAL, AND MISCELLANEOUS CAUSES OF DELIRIUM

II. Medications, Toxins, and Abused Substances
   A. Prescribed drugs—any drug affecting the brain, especially
      1. Sedatives, hypnotics, and tranquilizers
      2. Antidepressants
      3. Cimetidine and related drugs
      4. Narcotics
      5. Theophylline and related drugs
      6. Anticonvulsants
   B. Exogenous toxins
      1. Organophosphates
      2. Heavy metals
      3. Carbon monoxide
      4. Methanol, isopropyl alcohol
   C. Abused substances
      1. Alcohol (ethanol)
      2. Cocaine
      3. Amphetamines
      4. Narcotics and heroin
      5. Phencyclidine
      6. Hallucinogens—LSD, mescaline
      7. Toxic vapors—glue, toluene
   D. Withdrawal from abused substances, especially
      1. Alcohol
      2. Benzodiazepines

III. Infections
   A. Systemic
      1. Sepsis
      2. Bacterial endocarditis
      3. Occult focal infections—pneumonia, gallbladder or urinary tract, especially in the elderly
   B. Central nervous system
      1. Meningitis
      2. Encephalitis
      3. Brain abscess
      4. AIDS and related infections

IV. Brain Lesions
   A. Acute stroke
      1. Infarction in unusual locations, especially parietal, occipital, and frontal
      2. Subarachnoid hemorrhage
   B. Tumors
      1. Gliomas in frontal or temporal lobe
      2. Metastases
   C. Wernicke's encephalopathy
   D. Subdural hematoma
   E. Traumatic brain contusion

V. Miscellaneous Neurological and Psychiatric Disorders
   A. Nonconvulsive status epilepticus
   B. Postictal state
   C. Postconcussion
   D. Atypical depression or psychosis
   E. "ICU psychosis"

VI. Multifactorial Encephalopathies
   A. Advanced age with minor infectious, drug, or metabolic stresses
   B. Pre-existing dementia with psychological and medical stress
   C. Critical illness with multiple system failures
   D. Debilitated AIDS or cancer patients with multiple drugs and infections

TREATMENT OF THE DELIRIOUS PATIENT

Management of delirium addresses both the etiology and the cognitive–behavioral effects. Any reversible metabolic, toxic, infectious, or other cause must be treated promptly. The best general rule is to treat all disordered medical conditions, attempting to restore the brain's metabolic and physiologic environment to normal. At the same time, all drugs with any possible CNS effect should be discontinued if the medical situation allows.

Management of the symptoms of the encephalopathy usually addresses three issues: (1) safety of the patient and staff; (2) autonomic dysfunction; and (3) comfort measures. Delirious patients often have potentially dangerous behaviors: pulling out intravenous lines, endotracheal tubes, and catheters; climbing over bed side rails; and being physically violent. As a first step in management, the physician and nurses caring for the patient develop a coordinated plan for behavior control, including physical restraints and sedation. Delirious patients are often calmed by talking with them, frequent reassurance, reorientation, and firm instructions to stop dangerous activity. Placing the patient in a well-lit, quiet room with music from a bedside radio often helps. For violent and uncontrolled patients, gauze mittens, physical limb restraints, and a Posey belt can prevent harm to the patient and others.

Judicious use of medications is necessary in agitated, out-of-control patients. Haloperidol may be given orally or parenterally. Elderly patients may respond well to 0.5 mg twice/day. Men with drug-related or other violent delirium may require 30 mg or more in divided intravenous doses over several hours. Benzodiazepines are also valuable and are the drug of choice in alcohol and sedative drug-withdrawal delirium. The patient's age, weight, and clinical condition dictate the dose and route. Acute, severe delirium may require high doses of intravenous diazepam (30 mg or more total over 24 hours) or lorazepam (12 mg or more total in divided doses). Early high-dose oral or intravenous sedation is necessary in patients with known alcohol or drug withdrawal delirium to abort development of a more severe, medically dangerous condition.

Autonomic nervous system hyperactivity usually responds to adequate benzodiazepine sedation. Calcium-channel and catecholamine blocking agents have also been used in alcohol withdrawal. Adequate hydration is important. Many patients admitted with delirium are dehydrated, and diaphoresis often aggravates the situation. Thiamine must be given to all patients with suspected alcoholism (100 mg IV immediately and then 100 mg/day for 4 days).

Patient comfort measures rely on expert nursing care, including verbal reassurance and making the patient physically comfortable, especially if restrained. Frequent observation of restrained patients is also important for early detection and correction of restraint abrasions of the wrists and ankles. Repeated explanations to reorient the patient and engaging the patient in conversation help calm disordered behavior.

COMMON SPECIFIC ENCEPHALOPATHIES

Several discrete encephalopathies frequently cause delirium and should be considered in any confused patient.

REVERSIBLE ANOXIC ENCEPHALOPATHY

Reversible anoxic encephalopathy is commonly seen in patients with respiratory failure causing hypoxemia. Normal mental function usually returns promptly and completely with restoration of normal arterial oxygen content.

POSTANOXIC ENCEPHALOPATHY

The more difficult case is that of postanoxic encephalopathy. Severe hypoxia or global brain ischemia for several minutes leads to prolonged brain dysfunction.[2, 13] Common causes are cardiac arrest, respiratory arrest, anesthetic accidents, and strangulation. After the acute event, the patient usually is unconscious, and the duration of the coma is proportional to the intensity and duration of the initial insult. As the patient awakens, there remains an encephalopathy, usually characterized by severe retrograde and anterograde amnesia, plus global confusion. The time period included in the amnesia later contracts, stabilizing after several days. During the encephalopathy, the patient also has marked difficulty establishing new memories. Frequently, patients suffer from a permanent residual dementia, with prominent deficits of memory functions.[14] The most reliable clinical marker of permanent brain dysfunction is duration of postevent unconsciousness. Many therapies have failed to prevent or reverse postanoxic encephalopathy, including corticosteroids, hyperbaric oxygenation, high-dose barbiturates, and calcium-channel blocking agents.[15, 16] The best treatment is prevention or prompt reversal of the initial hypoxic-ischemic event.

MYOCLONIC STATUS EPILEPTICUS

A particularly ominous acute complication of anoxic encephalopathy is repetitive myoclonic jerks combined with generalized seizures. These can be almost continuous, a situation called *myoclonic status epilepticus*.[17] Treatment is usually ineffective, probably because the condition is a marker for severe, irreversible neuronal injury. High-dose intravenous phenytoin, benzodiazepines, and barbiturates can be tried. Valproic acid given by nasogastric tube or by enema may be helpful in rare cases.

HEPATIC ENCEPHALOPATHY

Hepatic encephalopathy is a prototypical metabolic encephalopathy.[6, 18] It usually presents as an apathetic, quietly confused patient who has known chronic liver disease. More severe cases progress to coma, severe systemic medical complications, and death. The mechanism of brain dysfunction in hepatic failure probably is multifactorial. Excessive blood and brain ammonia, elevated brain γ-aminobutyric acid, false neurotransmitters, endogenous benzodiazepine-like substances, and abnormal fatty acid metabolism have all been implicated, but none definitively.[6, 18] Diagnosis of hepatic encephalopathy is usually based on the history, clinical signs, and laboratory findings of severe hepatic disease. There is no single diagnostic test. Elevated blood ammonia level in a properly collected, promptly tested arterial blood specimen is a helpful finding, but normal blood ammonia does not rule out liver failure.[6] Another suggestive finding is the presence of bifrontal triphasic complexes on the EEG.[12] However, most patients with hepatic encephalopathy have only nonspecific, diffuse slowing and disorganization of the brain activity, and other metabolic conditions occasionally cause triphasic waves. A common metabolic finding on arterial blood gas testing is respiratory alkalosis.

Treatment begins with reversal of precipitating medical conditions—commonly gastrointestinal bleeding, systemic infections, and electrolyte imbalance.[6, 18] Clearing the intestine of blood and ammonia-producing bacteria is accomplished with lactulose (20 to 30 g by mouth three to four times/day) and enemas. Neomycin (2 to 6 g by mouth per day in divided doses) may help by reducing toxin-producing intestinal bacteria. The patient should be placed on a low-protein diet, and optimal fluid and electrolyte balance should be maintained with intravenous therapy. Multivitamin supplements, thiamine, and vitamin K are important adjunctive treatments.

UREMIC ENCEPHALOPATHY

Renal failure can lead to a typical delirium.[6, 19] Clinical features are not diagnostically distinct but, more commonly than other metabolic encephalopathies, include multifocal myoclonus and seizures.[19] The pathophysiology of uremic encephalopathy is even less understood than of liver failure. Again, probably multiple toxic and metabolic factors contribute to brain dysfunction. The diagnosis rests on clinical and laboratory findings of renal failure. Treatment depends on reversal of the renal disease and the associated metabolic disturbances, plus dialysis, when indicated.

Rapid dialysis itself can induce a syndrome of headache, delirium, cramps, and convulsions—the *dialysis disequilibrium syndrome*.[6, 20] This probably is due to water shifting into the brain during dialysis, causing brain edema.

GLUCOSE-RELATED ENCEPHALOPATHY

Glucose-related encephalopathies are usually easily recognized because of typical clinical settings and diagnostic laboratory findings. Hypoglycemia is recognized and treated so easily that it rarely presents a problem for the ICU physician.[21] Diabetic ketoacidosis likewise is a common but readily managed cause of acute confusion.[6, 22] Brain function returns to baseline once the ketoacidosis has cleared. The nonketotic, hyperglycemic, hyperosmolar state is a less commonly recognized cause of encephalopathy.[6, 23] Unusual neurological features of hyperosmolar encephalopathy include focal and continuous focal seizures (*epilepsia partialis continua*), and choreoathetosis.[24]

INTOXICATION-INDUCED ENCEPHALOPATHY

Acute intoxication is a frequent, usually easily recognized and treated cause of encephalopathy with delirium. In Colorado in 1989, the most common intoxicants requiring hospitalization were antidepressants (12.7 percent), benzodiazepines (12.0 percent), aspirin (8.6 percent), and ethanol (6.7 percent), followed by carbon monoxide and pesticides.[25] High case fatality rates were caused by asthma medications, cardiac glycosides, antiarrhythmics, and carbon monoxide.

Management of acute intoxication begins with life support, including intubation as necessary, and immediate administration of specific antidotes if the toxin is known. Generic principles of management include recovery of unabsorbed toxins by gastric lavage, reduction of absorption of toxin by administering activated charcoal by orogastric tube, and accelerating elimination of toxin using cathartics (Table 1-2).[26] Other methods of accelerating blood clearance of some toxins include forced diuresis, alkalinization of the urine, peritoneal or hemodialysis, hemoperfusion, and hemofiltration.[27] Early consultations with a clinical toxicologist, regional poison center, and toxicology texts are valuable in guiding specific management.

Table 1-2. EARLY STEPS IN MANAGEMENT OF DRUG OVERDOSE[a]

Intubation: any patient with depression of consciousness

Gastric lavage: room temperature normal saline in 200-ml aliquots via large-bore orogastric tube. Administer several liters until return is clear

Activated charcoal: 1 g/kg body weight by orogastric tube (maximum 100 g)

Cathartic: magnesium sulfate (250 mg/kg), magnesium citrate (4 ml/kg), or sorbitol (750 mg/kg)

[a] Size of tube, volumes, and doses must be reduced for children. Each step has specific contraindications (e.g., large ingestions of acids or intestinal obstruction).[26]

DRUG WITHDRAWAL DELIRIUM

Drug withdrawal is a common cause of delirium in public inner-city hospitals. The most common drug is ethanol. Any ICU patient with agitation and psychomotor hyperactivity should be considered for alcohol or other drug withdrawal. Common drugs other than alcohol are benzodiazepines and hypnotics.

The classic features of a drug withdrawal delirium are hypervigilance, excessive motor activity, rambling—even boisterous—speech, disordered sleep–wake cycle, and prominent autonomic dysfunction, usually seen as tachycardia and hypertension. More severe delirium includes sensory misperceptions, delusions, and hallucinations, usually poorly formed, frightening visual images.

Definitive diagnosis is made based on history of alcohol or other drug use, recent abstinence, and a thorough clinical work-up to exclude other causes. Important "rule-outs" are acute drug intoxication, especially cocaine, amphetamines, and PCP, as well as CNS infection, especially meningitis.

MEDICATION-INDUCED ENCEPHALOPATHY

Medications, both physician-prescribed and the over-the-counter variety, are common causes of delirium. Particularly susceptible to medication-induced encephalopathy are elderly, demented, or retarded patients and patients with pre-existing brain disorders, such as stroke, Parkinson's disease, multiple sclerosis, and trauma. Common medications usually not associated with delirium but which can cause delirium in occasional cases are aspirin, antihypertensive agents, antidepressants, anticonvulsants, corticosteroids, nonsteroidal anti-inflammatory agents, digoxin, calcium-channel blockers, H_2-receptor antagonists, over-the-counter "cold pills," and any medication with anticholinergic properties.[28]

METABOLIC ENCEPHALOPATHIES IN CHILDREN

Children are prone to the same acute metabolic encephalopathies as adults. However, inborn errors of metabolism are more likely to first appear in childhood. Some problems are unique to children, such as the complications of prematurity or of the birth process. Premature infants may develop coma as a result of intraventricular hemorrhage.[29] Newborns of all gestational ages may develop alterations of consciousness as a result of neonatal hypoxic-ischemic encephalopathy. This condition is often attributable to events preceding the actual delivery, sometimes by weeks or months. In cases of suspected neonatal hypoxic-ischemic encephalopathy, a thorough search for factors interfering with normal gestation should be made, although such factors are frequently difficult to identify.

Reye syndrome has received much attention in the pediatric literature. This disorder often follows a viral illness and produces severe vomiting, followed by a declining level of consciousness and cerebral edema, which may be lethal. Laboratory abnormalities include hypoglycemia and abnormal liver function tests. The CNS dysfunction of Reye syndrome is not secondary to hepatic dysfunction, but rather represents a primary component of the illness, most likely a generalized mitochondrial dysfunction. Some epidemiologic evidence suggests an association between aspirin use and the development of Reye syndrome, but a convincing biochemical link has not been shown. Although the cause of Reye syndrome is unclear, some defined metabolic disorders have been identified as causes of the syndrome. All cases of Reye syndrome should be investigated vigorously for a possible underlying inborn error of metabolism, especially in cases of recurrent or familial Reye syndrome. Treatment of Reye syndrome is directed toward reversal of any identifiable underlying metabolic disorder, administration of glucose, and management of increased intracranial pressure. Corticosteroids have been advocated, but are not of proven benefit.

The inborn errors of metabolism that commonly produce acute encephalopathy are disorders of glucose metabolism or of organic acid metabolism.[30] These children may have remarkably focal neurological findings, and the presence of such findings should not exclude consideration of an inborn error. Most of these disorders do not have diagnostic clinical features, so the diagnosis is usually made on biochemical grounds. An exception is nonketotic hyperglycinemia, one of the few causes of encephalopathy with prominent myoclonus in childhood. Elevations of glycine may be demonstrable only in the cerebrospinal fluid, and this diagnosis cannot be excluded on the basis of normal serum glycine levels alone.

An unexplained, rapidly deteriorating level of consciousness, particularly if episodic or if occurring in a child with unexplained developmental delay or with a family history of metabolic disease, should alert the clinician to the possibility of an inborn error of metabolism. Unexplained fetal or early childhood death in siblings should also suggest the need for a metabolic evaluation. Acute encephalopathy caused by an inborn error of metabolism often, but not invariably, leads to a metabolic acidosis that can be detected by the usual tests.

The general laboratory approach to a child in whom a primary metabolic disorder is suspected usually includes measurement of serum bicarbonate, glucose, ammonia, amino acids, and urine organic acids. Measurement of serum lactate and pyruvate is indicated when a mitochondrial defect is suspected.[31] Measurement of octanoylcarnitine is useful in diagnosing medium-chain acylCoA dehydrogenase deficiency—a fairly common cause of relapsing childhood encephalopathy. This disorder is often episodic, leaving the child normal between episodes. It may not appear until late in childhood or even the teenage years.

Treatment of this group of disorders is aimed at reversal of all metabolic abnormalities (hypoglycemia, acidosis, etc.), control of increased intracranial pressure, and reversal of the primary defect, if possible. Some specific treatments are available (e.g., vitamin B_{12} administration in some cases of methylmalonic acidemia). Consultation with a clinician experienced in diagnosis and management of these childhood disorders is recommended.

DIAGNOSIS AND MANAGEMENT OF COMA IN THE MEDICAL ICU

Coma is best defined as eyes-closed unresponsiveness caused by a disorder of the brain. However, coma is only a portion of the broad spectrum of impairment of consciousness (alertness), ranging from slight drowsiness to clinical brain death.[2] For this discussion, the focus is on patients in coma. The principles of management of the comatose patient are to (1) provide life support, (2) preserve brain function, (3) define and treat the cause, (4) prevent medical complications, and (5) follow the patient's neurological and medical signs closely until the patient awakens.[32]

The immediate steps in managing a comatose patient include intubation to control the airway and prevent aspiration, establishing an intravenous line to administer fluids and drugs, and inserting a urinary catheter to monitor output.[32] Any suspicion of hypoventilation prompts arterial blood gas testing and the institution of mechanical ventilation. Preservation of brain function is ensured by the presumptive administration of oxygen and, when clinically indicated, intravenous boluses of glucose (50 ml of 50 percent dextrose in water for adults) and a narcotic antagonist (naloxone, 1.0 mg IV), followed by repeat doses if a partial response is obtained initially. A thiamine bolus of 100 mg should be given to malnourished or suspected alcoholic patients.

Defining the cause of coma demands all the skills of a clinician—a thorough history, detailed medical and neurological examinations, and thoughtful use of laboratory tests. A guiding principle in early management is to search for historic and examination clues suggesting an intracranial mass lesion. If the clues are present, an emergency CT scan of the head is required to diagnose the lesion and guide immediate decisions about surgery, treatment of intracranial pressure, and management of blood pressure and fluids. The clues suggesting possible intracranial mass are listed in Table 1-3. If no mass is suspected, or mass is ruled out by CT scan, a lumbar puncture should be performed to look for CNS infection or blood. Bacterial, tuberculous, and fungal meningitis, herpes simplex encephalitis, and occult subarachnoid hemorrhage can present as coma with few meningeal signs, especially in AIDS, immunosuppressed, and elderly patients.

Table 1-3. CLUES SUGGESTING POSSIBLE INTRACRANIAL MASS

History: trauma, focal neurological symptoms (e.g., arm or leg weakness), known cancer, alcoholism, bleeding disorder, anticoagulant treatment, recent sinusitis

General examination: hypertension (suggests increased intracranial pressure), bradycardia, signs of trauma, bleeding, cancer, or infection

Neurological examination: papilledema, asymmetric pupils, eye movement, limb movement, limb posture or tendon reflexes, unilateral Babinski sign, diffusely hyperactive tendon reflexes

Laboratory tests are guided by the clinical history and findings and are the same as those recommended for work-up of the delirious patient.[2, 32] Definitive therapy follows a specific etiologic diagnosis.

Medical complications begin to occur within hours of the onset of coma. Aspiration of oral secretions or regurgitated stomach contents cause aspiration pneumonia. Partially open, unblinking eyes lead to conjunctivitis and corneal abrasions. Patients lying in one position develop pulmonary atelectasis, skin ulcerations, and joint contractures. Indwelling catheters promote urinary infections. Unmoving legs develop thrombophlebitis, sometimes causing pulmonary emboli. The physician's admission orders and the nursing care plan must address each of these potential complications. Daily rounds are focused to identify and treat any complication as early as possible.

The final principle of management requires repeated detailed observation of the patient's neurological signs to ensure they are improving. Modern ICUs use a bedside flow sheet to document and track the patient's vital signs, input, output, etc. Neurological signs should be part of the recorded observations of the comatose patient. Helpful observations include level of responsiveness, pupillary size, equality and reactivity, and movements of limbs when stimulated. A widely used measure of level of responsiveness is the Glasgow coma scale, which scores alertness based on verbal responses, motor activity, and eye opening to stimulation.[33, 34]

PROGNOSIS OF NONTRAUMATIC COMA

Clinical research in the last two decades has established the grave prognosis of patients in nontraumatic coma. One-year survival of such patients is about 12 percent when the coma lasts 6 hours or longer.[35] The main cause of death is the primary medical condition underlying the coma. There is no convincing evidence that intensive care has reduced medical coma's morbidity or mortality. To the contrary, there is some evidence that ICU care does not improve 30-day mortality.[35]

Predicting the outcome for an individual comatose patient is impossible, yet physicians must make clinical decisions and communicate with families based on some estimate of outcome. Data are not yet complete enough to guide rigorous predictions, but several clinical series provide some guidelines.[33–37] The authors' *rules of thumb* based on the literature and clinical experience in patients with medically caused coma are stated in Table 1-4. The best two references are those of Levy and associates.[35, 37]

Table 1-4. "RULES OF THUMB" FOR PROGNOSIS IN PATIENTS WITH MEDICAL COMA[a]

Good prognosis (i.e., will be normal or able to return to work or full self-care): patient awakens and is talking within hours of onset of coma

Bad outcome (i.e., very unlikely to return to independent living): patient with absent brainstem reflexes (i.e., pupillary light, corneal and caloric eye movement reflexes) at 24 hours

Indeterminate outcome (i.e., cannot predict): patients between the two above groups. Wait 48 hours. Then, level of alertness and verbal communication are best correlates of eventual outcome

Modifiers:
    Prognosis best in metabolic conditions, intermediate with hypoxic or global ischemic cause, and worst with cerebrovascular lesions
    Prognosis worse with advancing age
    Prognosis worse with prior brain lesion or disease
    Prognosis worse with multisystem or untreatable one-system disease

---

[a] Excluding drug overdoses.

REFERENCES

1. Lloyd GER: Hippocratic Writings. Penguin Classics Ed. Penguin Books, New York, 1978
2. Plum F, Posner J: The Diagnosis of Stupor and Coma. 3rd Ed. FA Davis, Philadelphia, 1980
3. Cameron DG, Thomas RI, Mulvihill M, Bronheim H: Delirium: a test of the Diagnostic and Statistical Manual III criteria on medical inpatients. J Am Geriatr Soc 35:1007, 1987

4. Francis J, Martin D, Kapoor WN: A prospective study of delirium in hospitalized elderly. JAMA 263:1097, 1990
5. Francis J, Kapoor WN: Delirium in hospitalized elderly. J Gen Intern Med 5:65, 1990
6. Lockwood AH: Toxic and metabolic encephalopathies. p. 1365. In Bradley WG, Daroff RB, Fenichel GM, Marsden CD (eds): Neurology in Clinical Practice. Butterworth-Heinemann, Boston, 1991
7. Folstein MF, Folstein SE, McHugh PR: "Mini-mental state": a practical method for grading the cognitive state of patients for the clinician. J Psychiatr Res 12:189, 1975
8. Schwamm LH, Van Dyke C, Kiernan RJ et al: The neurobehavioral cognitive status examination: comparison with the cognitive capacity screening examination and the mini-mental state examination in a neurosurgical population. Ann Intern Med 107:486, 1987
9. Inouye SK, Van Dyke CH, Alessi CA et al: Clarifying confusion: the confusion assessment method. Ann Intern Med 113:941, 1990
10. Leavitt S, Tyler HP: Studies in asterixis. Arch Neurol 10:360, 1964
11. Leehey M, Gilden D: Neurologic disorders associated with the HIV and HTLV-1 viruses. p. 1. In Appel SH (ed): Current Neurology. Vol. 10. Year Book Medical Publishers, Chicago, 1990
12. Brenner RP: The electroencephalogram in altered states of consciousness. Neurol Clin 3:615, 1985
13. Plum F, Pulsinelli WA: Cerebral metabolism and hypoxic-ischemic brain injury. p. 1086. In Asbury A, McKhann GM, McDonald WI (eds): Diseases of the Nervous System. Vol. II. Ardmore Medical Books, Philadelphia, 1988
14. Earnest MP, Yarnell PR, Merrill SL, Knapp GL: Long-term survival and neurologic status after resuscitation from out-of-hospital cardiac arrest. Neurology 30:1298, 1980
15. Brain Resuscitation Clinical Trial I Study Group: Randomized clinical study of thiopental loading in comatose survivors of cardiac arrest. N Engl J Med 314:397, 1986
16. Brain Resuscitation Clinical Trial II Study Group: A randomized clinical study of a calcium-entry blocker (lidoflazine) in the treatment of comatose survivors of cardiac arrest. N Engl J Med 324:1225, 1991
17. Jumao-as A, Brenner RP: Myoclonic status epilepticus: a clinical and electroencephalographic study. Neurology 40:1199, 1990
18. Fraser CL, Arieff AI: Hepatic encephalopathy. N Engl J Med 313:865, 1985
19. Raskin NH, Fishman RA: Neurologic disorders in renal failure (2 parts). N Engl J Med 294:143, 204, 1976
20. O'Hare JA, Callaghan NM, Murnaghan DJ: Dialysis encephalopathy—clinical, electroencephalographic and interventional aspects. Medicine 62:129, 1983
21. Malouf R, Brust JCM: Hypoglycemia: causes, neurological manifestations and outcome. Ann Neurol 17:421, 1985
22. Foster DW, McGarry JD: The metabolic derangements and treatment of diabetic ketoacidosis. N Engl J Med 309:159, 1983
23. Arieff AA, Carroll HJ: Nonketotic, hyperosmolar coma with hyperglycemia: clinical features, pathophysiology, renal function, acid–base balance, plasma–cerebrospinal fluid equilibria and the effects of therapy in 37 cases. Medicine 51:73, 1972
24. Singh BM, Strobos RJ: Epilepsia partialis continua associated with nonketotic hyperglycemia: clinical and biochemical profile of 21 patients. Ann Neurol 8:155, 1980
25. Doescher M: Hospitalizations for poisoning, Colorado—1989. p. 1. In Hoffman RE

(ed): Colorado Disease Bulletin. Vol. 18. Colorado Department of Health, Denver, 1991

26. Flomenbaum NE, Goldfrank LR, Weisman RS et al: General management of the poisoned or overdosed patient. p. 5. In Goldfrank LR, Weisman RS, Flomenbaum NE et al (eds): Goldfrank's Toxicologic Emergencies. 4th Ed. Appleton-Century-Crofts, East Norwalk, CT, 1990

27. Pond S: Principles of techniques used to enhance elimination of toxic compounds. p. 21. In Goldfrank LR, Weisman RS, Flomenbaum NE et al (eds): Goldfrank's Toxicologic Emergencies. 4th Ed. Appleton-Century-Crofts, East Norwalk, CT, 1990

28. Morrison RL, Katz IR: Drug-related cognitive impairment: current progress and recurrent problems. Ann Rev Gerontol Geriatr 9:232, 1989

29. Volpe JJ: Intraventricular hemorrhage in the premature infant—current concepts. Part II. Ann Neurol 25:109, 1989

30. Wraith JE: Diagnosis and management of inborn errors of metabolism. Arch Dis Child 64:1410, 1989

31. Applegarth DA, Dimmick JE, Toone JR: Laboratory detection of metabolic disease. Pediatr Clin North Am 36:49, 1989

32. Earnest MP, Cantrill SV: Coma. p. 1225. In Bayless TM, Brain MC, Cherniack RM (eds): Current Therapy in Internal Medicine. Vol. 2. BC Decker, Toronto, 1987

33. Sacco RL, VanGool R, Molvi JP, Hauser WA: Nontraumatic coma—Glasgow Coma Scale and coma etiology as predictors of 2-week outcome. Arch Neurol 47:1181, 1990

34. Mullie A, Verstringe P, Buylaert W et al: Predictive value of Glasgow Coma Score for awakening after out-of-hospital cardiac arrest. Lancet 1:137, 1988

35. Levy DE, Bates D, Caronna JJ et al: Prognosis in nontraumatic coma. Ann Intern Med 95:293, 1981

36. Earnest MP, Breckinridge JC, Yarnell PR, Oliva PB: Quality of survival after out-of-hospital cardiac arrest: predictive value of early neurologic evaluation. Neurology 29:59, 1979

37. Levy DE, Caronna JJ, Singer BH: Predicting outcome from hypoxic-ischemic coma. JAMA 253:1420, 1985

2

Acute Stroke

Sandra K. Hanson
James C. Grotta

Stroke is a major cause of death in acute care hospitals. About 500,000 new strokes occur yearly in the United States, and it is the third leading cause of death in almost all surveys. In Texas alone in 1990, there were 83,000 stroke deaths compared with 6,200 accidental deaths and 2,400 homicides. The mortality from stroke has declined steadily during the last 20 years, largely because of better control of hypertension, but a 25 percent rate of disability results in billions of dollars of health care expenditures and lost earnings. Risk factors for stroke are generally the same as those for coronary artery disease, although hypertension, atrial fibrillation, previous cerebrovascular symptoms, and carotid stenosis are particularly important. Diabetes, tobacco use, coronary artery disease, unfavorable lipid profile, and elevated fibrinogen have been identified as other important risks. Increasing age results in both more strokes and higher mortality.

Mortality after stroke averages approximately 15 percent with either carotid or vertebrobasilar distribution infarction but increases to 30 percent to 50 percent with supratentorial or infratentorial hemorrhage. Mortality from hemorrhage is almost entirely the result of increased intracranial pressure (ICP) and its consequences, and therefore depends on both the location and size of the hematoma. Most deaths from intracerebral hemorrhage occur during the first week. Cerebral infarction can also cause death because of cerebral swelling, although such swelling becomes maximal 3 to 5 days after the onset of symptoms and rarely during the first few hours. Pneumonia (often caused by silent aspiration), pulmonary embolism, and cardiac arrhythmias and myocardial infarction are other important causes of death in stroke patients (Fig. 2-1).[1]

Disability after a stroke increases with age and also with rising comorbidities (i.e., other illnesses, such as heart disease and arthritis). Different aspects of neurological dysfunction tend to recover at different rates. While neglect of the affected paralyzed side almost always completely recovers, it may last for up to 1 month after stroke and severely impair rehabilitative efforts. Motor

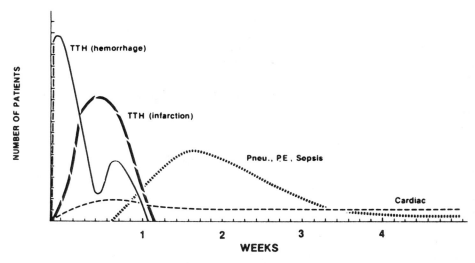

Fig. 2-1 Causes of death after cerebral infarction and hemorrhage and time course of their presentation. Abbreviations: TTH, transtentorial herniation; Pneu, pneumonia; PE, pulmonary embolus. (From Silver et al,[1] with permission.)

function and langauge function show variable amounts and rates of improvement. Patients seen early after stroke often show a worsening of their weakness and level of consciousness during the first 3 days and then a gradual improvement during the next month. In general, the greatest improvement in the neurological examination occurs over the first month, with further gradual improvement coming over a 6-month period. Although it is difficult to predict recovery during the acute phase of hospitalization, in general a patient with no recovery of function in an affected limb by 2 weeks is unlikely to regain normal function.

Although the amount of weakness clearly contributes to disability after stroke, the most important determinant of independent functioning after 6 months is the cognitive status of the patient. Language dysfunction, visual impairment, dementia, and depression can all result in greater dependency than severe paralysis.

This chapter provides the physician in the emergency department and the intensive care unit with enough information to properly evaluate and treat the acute stroke patient in order to minimize both mortality and morbidity. Recent studies have shown that stroke intensive care units can have a major impact, both on reducing mortality and improving functional outcome. In one recent study of patients randomly treated in a stroke intensive care unit versus a general medical ward, 6-week mortality was 7 percent in the stroke unit versus 17 percent in general medical ward patients, and the Barthel score, which measures the patient's ability to bathe, dress, and feed themselves and to ambulate, was 21 percent better in stroke unit patients.[2]

CLASSIFICATION OF STROKES

The term *stroke* usually applies to any sort of cerebrovascular disease, either ischemic or hemorrhagic, with either permanent or transient symptoms (Fig. 2-2).[3] Of patients presenting to an emergency department with focal neurological signs suggesting stroke, slightly more than 10 percent will turn out to have transient ischemic attacks (TIAs), with symptoms resolving within 24 hours. Some of these patients may have had a minor stroke, with radiographic evidence of infarction eventually showing up on computed tomography (CT) scan but no residual neurological deficit. As is discussed later, it is extremely important that patients with TIAs have a thorough evaluation and institution of appropriate therapy in order to prevent a subsequent disabling stroke. Of those patients admitted with permanent neurological deficit, approximately two-thirds will have a cerebral infarct and one-third will have a cerebral hemorrhage. This distinction may be extremely difficult to make on a clinical basis. Decreased level of consciousness within the first few hours of symptom onset is more suggestive of a cerebral hemorrhage because of the acute increase in ICP. CT scan immediately on arrival in the emergency department is the most reliable way to distinguish between infarct and hemorrhage, and should be carried out in any patient suspected of a stroke.

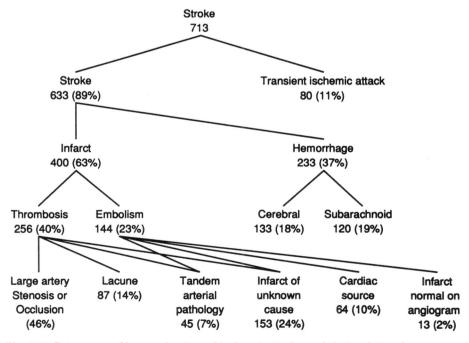

Fig. 2-2 Categories of hemorrhagic and ischemic stroke and their relative frequency of occurrence. (From Mohr and Sacco,[3] with permission.)

It has been our observation that when patients are seen within the first 2 or 3 hours of the onset of symptoms, there is a slightly higher representation of patients with cerebral hemorrhage. This is probably because patients with cerebral hemorrhage have a more dramatic onset of symptoms, with severe paralysis occurring abruptly, often associated with severe headache, vomiting, markedly elevated systolic blood pressure, and decreasing level of consciousness. Patients with cerebral infarction often have a more gradual or stepwise onset, and symptoms may actually resolve. Such fluctuations are rarely seen with cerebral hemorrhage. Among patients with cerebral hemorrhage (in the absence of trauma), about two-thirds are parenchymal and the other one-third represent subarachnoid bleeding.

Subarachnoid hemorrhage usually presents with a prominent headache. In many cases, headache is the only symptom; emergency department physicians should have a high degree of suspicion of subarachnoid hemorrhage in any patient with a severe headache without good explanation, particularly if it is associated with mild neck stiffness. In such cases, a CT scan with thin cuts through the basal cisterns may often reveal small amounts of subarachnoid bleeding. If there is any question, a lumbar puncture should be carried out, looking for blood that is not seen clearly on the CT scan. In more severe cases of subarachnoid hemorrhage, the patients will often have a decreased level of consciousness, but usually do not have prominent focal neurological signs on presentation unless there has been hemorrhage into the brain parenchyma as well. Most subarachnoid hemorrhages are due to ruptured saccular, or "berry," aneurysms. However, in approximately 20 percent of patients, no source of bleeding can be found. The bleeding in some of these cases may be due to minor trauma, drug abuse (particularly cocaine), or coagulopathy, but in many cases, no cause is found.

Parenchymal hematomas are most often due to rupture of small caliber arterioles in the basal ganglia, thalamus, cerebellum, or brain stem. Such vessels are prone to rupture from long-standing hypertension, drug abuse, or amyloid angiopathy in elderly individuals. Among those patients with cerebral hemorrhage due to cocaine abuse, it has recently been reported that hemorrhages are more common with the use of cocaine hydrochloride as opposed to alkaloidal, or crack, cocaine.[4]

The classification of ischemic stroke is even more complicated. Ischemic strokes classically are divided into thrombotic (two-thirds) and embolic (one-third). Although this distinction often cannot be made with certainty, a combination of clinical and laboratory features helps distinguish the two (Table 2-1).[5] The importance of making this distinction is that the focus of diagnostic studies and subsequent therapy to prevent recurrent stroke differ, as will be discussed later. While the two subtypes can present in the same fashion, thrombotic infarcts more frequently have a progressive onset, as opposed to the sudden onset of embolic strokes. Thrombotic strokes are more common in patients with multiple stroke risk factors, particularly hypertension, diabetes, and lipid disturbances, whereas embolic strokes are more common in patients with severe atherosclerosis at the carotid bifurcation or underlying

Table 2-1. CLINICAL AND DIAGNOSTIC CRITERIA SUGGESTING
CARDIOEMBOLIC STROKE

Clinical Criteria
1. May occur in any age group but more common in young adults
2. Often sudden onset but may be stepwise progression of fluctuating course of focal neurological symptoms
3. Usually no antecedent TIA in the same vascular territory
4. Evidence of previous strokes in other vascular territories
5. Evidence of systemic embolism
6. Abnormal cardiac examination, with findings compatible with a likely source for emboli
7. No large artery source for emboli found

Diagnostic Studies
1. CT or MRI may demonstrate bland or hemorrhagic infarction(s) in a cortical and/or subcortical arterial distribution
2. Arteriography, if performed, can demonstrate a branch artery occlusion but no larger artery, extracranial source
3. Cardiac evaluation (electrocardiogram, transthoracic or transesophageal two-dimensional echocardiography, contrast echocardiography, ultrafast cardiac CT, Holter monitoring) demonstrates a likely source of embolism
4. Carotid duplex ultrasound: absence of hemodynamically consequential carotid stenosis

(From Love and Biller,[5] with permission.)

cardiac disease, such as atrial fibrillation, valvular disease, or mural thrombus associated with cardiomyopathy or acute myocardial infarction. Finally, the location of the infarct as determined by CT or magnetic resonance imaging (MRI) can also be helpful. Embolic infarcts most commonly affect cortical regions because the emboli obstruct branches of the major cerebral arteries. Multiple cortical infarcts suggest a cardiac source of embolism. Thrombotic infarcts, however, are often associated with occlusion of vessels supplying subcortical regions, resulting in either tiny lacunar infarcts or larger subcortical infarcts affecting the internal capsule and deep white matter. One syndrome important to recognize is thrombosis of the basilar artery. Obstruction of the basilar artery by thrombosis can develop over the course of hours and, if complete, is usually fatal. When basilar artery thrombosis is suspected, usually on the basis of a neurological examination demonstrating bilateral corticospinal tract dysfunction, ataxia, and cranial nerve abnormalities, most clinicians would recommend emergency anticoagulation.

Besides atherothrombosis, atheroembolism from a carotid plaque, and cardioembolism, other causes of ischemic stroke have been recognized, particularly in younger patients (Table 2-2).[6] Diseases of the blood vessels include inflammatory conditions such as vasculitis, an obliterative arteriopathy known as moyamoya disease, and either spontaneous or post-traumatic arterial dissection. The first two conditions should be suspected in patients without the usual stroke risk factors and in patients with multifocal symptoms and signs. Dissection should be suspected in any patient with stroke after exertion or trauma or in any patient with ischemic stroke and severe head pain. These arteriopathies can be diagnosed only by high-quality arteriography. The importance of making these diagnoses is that therapy may be different from conventional stroke (i.e., immunosuppressants for vasculitis, surgical revascularization for moyamoya disease, and anticoagulation for dissection).

Coagulation disturbances can also underlie strokes. Sickle cell anemia is the prototypical hematologic disorder leading to arterial occlusion. Strokes have also been reported secondary to thrombocytosis and polycythemia. Hypercoaguable states due to circulating lupus anticoagulant and deficiencies of antithrombin III, protein S, and protein C have also been described. The importance of making these diagnoses is that they mandate correction of the underlying hematologic abnormality.

Finally, complicated migraine, a poorly understood condition associated with spasm of the intracerebral vessels, can produce focal neurological deficits and cerebral infarction in some cases. This diagnosis must be kept in mind, particularly in young women with unusual stroke presentations associated with headache. Appropriate intervention can stop the pain and prevent the neurological symptoms from developing into a complete infarction.

Table 2-2.   CONDITIONS ASSOCIATED WITH FOCAL
CEREBRAL ISCHEMIA

Vascular Disorders
    Atherosclerosis
    Fibromuscular dysplasia
    Inflammatory disorders
        Giant cell arteritis
        Systemic lupus erythematosus
        Polyarteritis nodosa
        Granulomatous angiitis
        Syphilitic arteritis
    Carotid or vertebral artery dissection
    Multiple progressive intracranial arterial occlusions (moyamoya disease)
    Lacunar infarction
    Migraine
    Venous or sinus thrombosis

Cardiac Disorders
    Mural thrombus
    Rheumatic heart disease
    Arrhythmias
    Endocarditis
    Mitral valve prolapse
    Paradoxic embolus
    Atrial myxoma
    Prosthetic heart valves

Hematologic Disorders
    Thrombocytosis
    Polycythemia
    Sickle cell disease
    Leukocytosis
    Hypercoagulable states

(From Simon et al,[6] with permission)

PEDIATRIC STROKE

Stroke in the pediatric population differs from that in the adult population and should be considered separately. Similar to the adult population, the most common presenting symptom in childhood is hemiplegia (with or without seizure), occurring in 91 percent of cases in a series reported by Dusser et al.[7] In contrast, because of the immaturity of the nervous system, stroke in the neonate is distinctly different, usually presenting with seizure only. The onset of their seizures is between 8 and 60 hours after birth. They are usually focal clonic seizures, but seizure manifestations may occasionally be multifocal or subtle (apnea, tonic deviation of the eyes, fluttering of the eyelids, pedaling movements, sucking, or chewing). The incidence of neonatal infarction in Barmada's autopsy series was as high as 5.4 percent,[8] and with the advent of CT and MRI, more ischemic disease is being recognized in neonates. However, cerebral infarcts (in those that survive) are often missed diagnoses in the neonatal period because of the subtle presentation. Many patients show no neurological abnormality on examination or have only subtle tone changes on the affected side. The reported outcome in neonatal stroke is variable. As children grow older, a spastic hemiplegia may become evident, or children may develop normally despite a sizable infarct.[9] In childhood stroke, several authors have reported high frequencies of residual motor deficit, ranging from 73 percent to 91 percent of patients.[10]

Although the etiology of ischemic stroke in childhood differs from that of the adult, it can be separated into similar categories to those described in the adult (i.e., disease of the carotid, cardioembolic sources, and alterations in blood rheology). Disease of the carotid would include the vasculopathies occurring in the younger age group. Moyamoya disease is a progressive occlusive disorder of the distal internal carotid artery and circle of Willis, occurring in children younger than 10 years, with a second peak incidence in adulthood. It follows a course of repeated episodes of transient ischemia and completed strokes in childhood but, in adults, will often present with hemorrhage. Other vasculopathies occurring in childhood and adolescence include fibromuscular dysplasia, Kawasaki disease, Takayasu's arteritis, hypersensitivity vasculitis, and systemic lupus erythematosus. A premature atheromatous process can occur in the young in the setting of familial hyperlipidemic disorders and in homocystinuria. Direct trauma to the carotid or vertebral arteries may result in dissection and subsequent thrombosis and stroke. This may be the result of trivial neck injury in sporting activities and with exercise. Perinatal traumatic vascular injury, with intimal damage and thrombus formation, has also been documented in the internal carotid and vertebral arteries.[11] In addition, the carotid may be injured via the tonsillar fossa during tonsillectomy or with a long, blunt object (such as a pencil) placed in the mouth. Another consideration should be stroke occurring as the result of drugs of abuse (cocaine, amphetamines). Bacterial meningitis is a common cause of both arterial and venous infarctions in infancy and childhood.

Cardioembolic stroke occurs in the setting of congenital heart disease, rheumatic heart disease, and with mitral valve prolapse. Children with the cyanotic congenital heart diseases are particularly prone to developing cardioembolic problems. Venous sinus occlusion occurs in infants and is related to congestive heart failure and polycythemia, whereas arterial embolic occlusion tends to occur in children. In a series of children with stroke reported by Dusser et al,[7] 8 of 14 cases had cardiac disease. The cardiac disorders included double outlet/single ventricle, tetralogy of Fallot, transposition of the great vessels, pulmonary artery atresia, mitral stenosis, subacute bacterial endocarditis, and supraventricular tachycardia.[7] Mitral valve prolapse occurs in 5 percent of all children, but is a rare cause of recurrent attacks of ischemia.[12] An additional consideration in the neonatal population includes embolization of placental tissue via a patent ductus arteriosus.

Disorders of coagulation or blood rheology are also part of the differential in children. Hypercoagulable states can be produced by disseminated intravascular coagulation or with hereditary deficiencies of protein C, protein S, or antithrombin III, as in the adult population. Cancer is an important cause of stroke, which occurs in 4 percent of children with cancer.[13] The lymphoreticular disorders are the most common association. Common mechanisms for stroke with cancers include vascular thrombosis with disseminated intravascular coagulation, arterial or sagittal sinus thrombosis due to L-asparaginase therapy, infarction related to methotrexate therapy, sinus thrombosis due to metastatic neuroblastoma, and radiation-induced accelerated atherosclerosis. Sickle cell anemia can result in cerebral ischemia in childhood, with neurological complications occurring in 25 percent of homozygotes. Altered blood rheology with a decrease in total, hemispheral, or regional blood flow has been described.[14]

The constellation of mitochondrial myopathy, encephalopathy, lactic acidosis, and stroke-like episodes (MELAS) is an unusual cause of stroke in childhood. The children are normal at birth, but manifest a progressive course of growth retardation, deafness, seizures, strokes, myopathy, encephalopathy, and eventual coma.[15] There is no treatment for this disorder.

For many pediatric cases of stroke, no etiology can be identified. In the series of Dusser et al[7] of 44 patients with ischemic stroke, one-half had no identifiable reason for their events. In their patients with idiopathic stroke, there were no recurrences over an average follow-up period of 4 years. This is in stark contrast to those with cardiac disease or moyamoya disease.

DIAGNOSTIC STUDIES

The purposes of diagnostic studies after acute stroke are to determine the type of stroke and its probable etiology and to detect complications.

Stroke type can be determined largely on the basis of the history, neurological examination, and results of neuroimaging studies. The most commonly performed is a CT scan. Because of its high reliability in distinguishing cerebral hemorrhage from infarction, a noncontrast CT should be performed in all patients with stroke as soon as possible. This distinction is important before using antiplatelet or anticoagulation therapy and to detect and determine the extent of any mass effect from a hematoma. Finally, the management of blood pressure often differs in patients with acute hemorrhage versus infarction (*vide infra*). Among patients with cerebral infarcts, the CT scan is often normal in the first few hours but usually will show abnormalities after 12 or more hours. A repeat CT or MRI scan can help localize the infarct after this time. Patients with atypical presentations or those with unusual CT patterns should have a contrast-enhanced CT scan or MRI scan to exclude a tumor.

Once the determination has been made between cerebral infarct and hemorrhage, further evaluation is indicated to determine the etiology. In patients with intracerebral hemorrhage, ultimately a CT scan with contrast, MRI scan, or arteriogram should be performed to search for an underlying vascular malformation. Associated subarachnoid blood or suspicious areas on contrast CT or MRI increase the likelihood of finding an underlying malformation in patients with hemorrhage into one of the lobes of the brain.[16] Patients with subarachnoid hemorrhage should have an arteriogram as soon as possible to detect the source of bleeding, usually a saccular aneurysm. The arteriogram should be carried out within the first 24 to 48 hours, since taking the patient to surgery for definitive clipping of the aneurysm within the first 72 hours may help reduce morbidity and mortality from rebleeding. Furthermore, angiography after this time may be less likely to reveal the aneurysm because of intervening vasospasm, which occurs after 3 days. Transcranial Doppler ultrasound has largely replaced angiography for detecting and following the development of vasospasm in patients with subarachnoid hemorrhage.

Patients with clinical criteria suggesting cardioembolic stroke should have a two-dimensional echocardiogram and Holter monitor. If the two-dimensional echocardiogram is equivocal or a cardiac source is strongly suspected despite a negative two-dimensional echocardiogram, a transesophageal echocardiogram may detect an abnormality. A Holter monitor, or other method of cardiac monitoring, may detect an occult arrhythmia, particularly intermittent atrial fibrillation.

Carotid ultrasound and other noninvasive means of imaging the extracranial carotid circulation (such as MR angiography) are commonly ordered in acute ischemic stroke patients to detect severe occlusive disease. Because carotid endarterectomy has been proved effective for prevention of subsequent stroke in patients with TIAs or minor stroke associated with 70 percent or greater carotid stenosis, careful evaluation of the extracranial carotid arteries is indicated in all patients with carotid distribution stroke who are left with mild or no neurological deficit. In patients who are not candidates for surgery, these tests can still provide useful information about the status of the extracranial vessels. Patients with severe carotid stenosis and an unstable neurological picture might be candidates for acute anticoagulation therapy, and are also particularly vulnerable to downward fluctuations in blood pressure. Transcranial Doppler ultrasound is commonly used to evaluate the more distal circulation by insonating the vessels in the circle of Willis. At the present time, the reliability of this test to detect occlusive disease is variable.

Arteriography should be carried out in patients with severe carotid stenosis on ultrasound who are considered candidates for carotid endarterectomy and in patients with unusual presentations. These would include patients with a clinical syndrome suggestive of arterial dissection, patients with multiple infarcts suggestive of vasculitis, or progressing stroke suggestive of high-grade stenosis of an intracranial vessel. Arteriography in such patients is used to confirm the diagnosis prior to institution of therapy. It is possible that MR angiography will help limit the number of arteriograms carried out for these conditions. MRI can also produce useful information in these patients and is the imaging procedure of choice for detecting cerebral venous occlusion.

Certain blood studies should be carried out in all stroke patients, including complete blood cell count, differential blood cell count, platelets, prothrombin time, partial thromboplastin time, creatinine level, electrolytes, and blood glucose level. The blood glucose level is particularly important because hypoglycemia can be associated with focal neurological signs resembling a stroke. Other blood studies, such as detailed testing of the coagulation system by protein S, protein C, and antithrombin III levels, lupus anticoagulant and anticardiolipin antibody, connective tissue disease screen, and syphilis serology, may be indicated depending on the clinical situation. Serum cholesterol, low-density lipoprotein, high-density lipoprotein, and triglycerides should be measured in all patients with stroke but are unreliable in the acute setting. Fasting lipid profiles should be obtained once patients are on a stable diet and beyond the acute stroke phase.

An electrocardiogram should be obtained in all patients. A chest x-ray is a good idea in most patients, particularly smokers, those without a recent chest x-ray, and patients with severe stroke. A baseline chest x-ray may be valuable for comparison if the patient develops clinical evidence of aspiration pneumonia. Lumbar puncture is no longer carried out routinely in stroke patients. It should be performed to detect subarachnoid blood if this is suspected but not conclusively shown on CT scan, and in anyone in whom meningitis or some other inflammatory condition is suspected. It should be kept in mind that syphilis, acquired immunodeficiency syndrome, Lyme disease, and other more "occult" infections may underlie stroke, particularly in patients with systemic illness.

Measurements of cerebral blood flow are mostly used for clinical research purposes in the setting of acute ischemic stroke and not routinely used for patient management. Many techniques measure cerebral blood flow, including single photon emission computed tomography (SPECT), stable xenon-enhanced CT scanning, isotopic xenon, and positron emission tomography. New MRI protocols may soon be available for measuring cerebral blood flow. In the first few hours after ischemic stroke, cerebral blood flow correlates well with neurological deficit and ultimate outcome. However, arterial obstructions often fragment and are dissolved by endogenous thrombolytic mechanisms within the first 48 hours. Such spontaneous reperfusion will result in normal or even increased perfusion to destroyed tissue. In some cases, this reperfusion can be harmful, resulting in cerebral edema or hemorrhage. At this point, cerebral blood flow has little or no correlation with outcome. We have used cerebral blood flow measurements to help understand the time course of spontaneous reperfusion and the success of different reperfusion therapies, in particular thrombolysis.

In some patients with severe carotid or intracranial stenosis, cerebral blood flow measurements may be useful to help identify a chronic state of low perfusion, which may be ameliorated by appropriate surgical or medical therapy. The use of acetazolamide (Diamox) results in dilation of vessels in normally perfused areas. In ischemic regions, vessels are already maximally dilated and will not respond to Diamox. Consequently, comparing pre- and post-Diamox blood flow studies can help identify such low-flow regions.

MANAGEMENT

All patients with strokes should be admitted to the hospital.

TRANSIENT ISCHEMIC ATTACK

Patients with TIAs who recover completely prior to or after arrival in the emergency department still require careful evaluation and should probably be admitted to the hospital, if only overnight. The incidence of stroke after TIA may be as high as 20 percent to 25 percent in the first year, with the highest incidence in the first month or so. Multiple TIAs, carotid as opposed to retinal distribution events, and high-grade carotid stenosis all increase the risk of early subsequent stroke. Because of the proven efficacy of carotid endarterectomy and appropriate medical therapy, patients should be evaluated rapidly so that these therapies can be started. Studies of aspirin in patients with TIAs have shown that 1,300 mg daily reduces the risk of stroke. Analysis of all trials carried out to date indicates that doses as low as 300 mg are equally effective and result in approximately 20 percent risk reduction.[17] The efficacy of doses less than 300 mg/day, although effective for preventing myocardial infarction, has not been conclusively proven for stroke prevention, although they clearly are better tolerated than higher doses. Ticlopidine has recently been approved for stroke prevention. This drug is approximately 20 percent more effective than aspirin for stroke prevention.[18] Unfortunately, ticlopidine causes gastrointestinal intolerance in up to 20 percent of patients, and approximately 1 percent develop a reversible neutropenia. Consequently, patients must have blood counts every 2 weeks for the first 3 months of therapy with ticlopidine. The drug will be most useful for those patients intolerant of aspirin, those who continue to have symptoms while on aspirin, and those who are at particularly high risk because of multiple risk factors.[19]

Recently, carotid endarterectomy has been proved to dramatically reduce the incidence of stroke in symptomatic patients with 70 percent or greater stenosis of the appropriate internal carotid artery.[20] This assumes that patients will have surgery by experienced surgeons, with an operative risk of no greater than 4 percent to 5 percent, and that the narrowing is carefully documented by appropriate arteriography. All patients with carotid distribution TIAs should therefore be rapidly evaluated for the presence of carotid stenosis by ultrasound, MR angiography, or conventional arteriography.

GENERAL MANAGEMENT

In patients with completed strokes, careful attention to certain vital signs can reduce mortality and morbidity. These vital signs for stroke include blood pressure, intravascular volume, temperature, oxygenation, and blood glucose level.

Blood pressure management is the single most important variable in the emergency care of stroke patients. Normally, cerebral blood flow is autoregulated, so that wide fluctuations in blood pressure are tolerated without substantial change in cerebral perfusion. However, in the injured brain, the ability to autoregulate is lost, so that cerebral blood flow passively follows mean arterial blood pressure. Furthermore, in hypertensive patients, the autoregulatory curve is shifted upward so that cerebral blood flow begins to fall at a higher mean arterial blood pressure. Therefore, in patients with acute cerebral infarction, blood pressure should be lowered cautiously, if at all. If antihypertensive drugs are started, it would be best to monitor cerebral blood flow, but this is generally impossible. Aggressive reduction of blood pressure with parenteral drugs is indicated only in the setting of acute cerebral hemorrhage or in patients with cerebral infarction who are in danger of myocardial or renal damage from accelerated hypertension. In these cases, the best drug is either a parenteral β-blocker such as labetalol or a constant infusion of nitroprusside. The advantage of nitroprusside is that blood pressure can be carefully titrated to a desired level; the disadvantage is that this drug is a cerebral vasodilator, and may result in increased ICP in patients who already have mass effect from a hematoma or cerebral swelling. In patients with cerebral infarction and moderate hypertension (systolic blood pressure between 170 and 220 mmHg and diastolic pressures between 90 and 120 mmHg), we generally recommend withholding antihypertensive therapy in the emergency department. Often, the blood pressure will fall when the patient is moved to a quieter room, the bladder is emptied, and the patient is allowed to rest. If the blood pressure remains elevated, we will then generally lower the mean arterial blood pressure gradually by approximately 15 percent using oral therapy with an angiotensin-converting enzyme inhibitor such as captopril or a calcium antagonist such as nicardipine. We avoid sublingual use of calcium antagonists because of their rapid absorption and sometimes precipitous decline in blood pressure. We also avoid chronic use of centrally acting drugs such as β-blockers, clonidine, and reserpine. Whenever antihypertensive therapy is used, the patient should be carefully monitored so that therapy can be discontinued if there is any neurological deterioration.

In a series of nine patients receiving Swan-Ganz catheterization after acute ischemic stroke, volume depletion was detected in one-third, with pulmonary wedge pressures ranging from 1 to 11 mmHg (mean, 6.3 ± 3.5 mmHg).[21]

Volume expansion with hydroxyethyl starch resulted in an immediate increase in cardiac output. Aggressive volume expansion therapy and hemodilution have not been shown to be effective in acute stroke, and may result in increased cerebral edema and decreased oxygen delivery, respectively. However, correction of hypovolemia and optimization of cardiac output should be an important priority during the first few hours after admission.

Brain temperature has emerged as an extremely important variable in experimental studies of cerebral ischemia. Hypothermia substantially reduces infarct size, while hyperthermia increases the amount of damage. Up to one-third of stroke patients have had a preceding infectious illness,[22] and because aspiration pneumonia and pulmonary embolism commonly complicate stroke, fever should be carefully sought out and treated with appropriate antipyretic agents.

Tissue oxygenation is also vitally important in the management of stroke patients. Hypoxia will result in anaerobic metabolism, with greater production of damaging lactate and hydrogen ions, as well as depletion of energy stores needed for maintaining normal ionic gradients across neuronal membranes. The most common causes of hypoxia in stroke patients include aspiration pneumonia, pulmonary embolism, and congestive heart failure. Aspiration commonly results from inappropriately accelerated oral feeding. All patients with brainstem strokes and those with large hemispheric strokes may have impaired swallowing. All stroke patients should be carefully evaluated prior to the initiation of oral feedings. Because it is important to maintain adequate nutritional status, if a patient's swallowing ability has not returned after the first few days, a Dobbhoff tube or percutaneous gastrojejunostomy should be used, even if it is anticipated that the patient's ability to swallow will ultimately return. Speech pathologists and dietitians can provide invaluable help assessing the swallowing and nutritional status of stroke patients.

Subcutaneous heparin should be used in immobilized stroke patients to prevent deep venous thrombosis and pulmonary embolism, even in the presence of intracerebral hemorrhage; 5,000 units subcutaneously every 12 hours is the conventional dose. Pneumatic compression devices may be an alternative, particularly in patients with cerebral hemorrhage.

Patients with stroke often have obstructive breathing patterns, particularly when asleep, resulting in arterial oxygen desaturation. We routinely monitor the oxygenation of patients when they are sleeping and provide supplemental oxygen if desaturation occurs.

Blood glucose level is the final vital sign in stroke patients. Both hypoglycemia and hyperglycemia may be damaging to the injured brain. Hyperglycemia (>155 mg/dl) increases infarct size in experimental stroke models, and may result in worse outcome in clinical studies.[23] We therefore recommend that blood glucose levels substantially above this be treated with insulin.

Because of the importance of monitoring these vital signs, a dedicated stroke unit can reduce mortality and morbidity. There is no strict definition as to what constitutes such a unit. The most important consideration is that nursing and other personnel be trained to observe patients carefully, so that fluctuations in neurological status can be recognized, and to adhere to the general principles listed above. The importance of physical and occupational therapists, speech pathologists, nutritionists, and social workers in preventing and treating contractures, physiologic deconditioning, nutritional deficiencies, and depression is vital and can result in substantially improved outcome.

INCREASED INTRACRANIAL PRESSURE

The management of increased ICP in general will be addressed in Chapter 4. In stroke patients, problems with ICP occur most commonly after intracerebral hemorrhage but can also occur 2 to 4 days after massive infarction of either the cerebral or cerebellar hemisphere. The magnitude of the clinical problem from increased ICP depends almost entirely on the size of the hematoma and the residual space available for expansion, which depends on any pre-existing atrophy. For this reason, younger patients are often less tolerant of cerebral swelling than expected compared with older patients. Intracerebral hemorrhages can enlarge up to 30 percent to 50 percent during the first 24 hours.[24] It is sometimes unclear whether this enlargement is due to further bleeding or swelling within the hematoma. Significant hypertension should be controlled during the first 24 hours after cerebral hemorrhage. Sustained hypertension, which is a consequence of increased ICP, is best treated by lowering ICP. Aggressive lowering of blood pressure in the setting of increased ICP should only be carried out once adequate cerebral perfusion is ensured.

The indications for surgical decompression of hematomas are widely debated, and some authorities believe that surgery improves outcome on only rare occasions. A clinical trial is badly needed. In our experience with patients presenting within 6 hours of supratentorial hemorrhage, most awake patients with hematomas smaller than 3 cm in diameter or 20 cm^3 in volume and without extension of bleeding into the ventricles do reasonably well with conservative management and should not be exposed to surgery. On the other hand, comatose patients with hematomas larger than 5 cm in diameter or 50 cm^3 volume can be predicted to die or be left severely disabled, and are unlikely to benefit from aggressive treatment. Surgery might best be reserved for patients between these extremes. Careful observation of the patient and serial CT scans are important. Timely evacuation of cerebellar and lobar hematomas are more likely to improve outcome than with deeper putamenal or thalamic hematomas. Stereotactic aspiration may be an alternative for these deeper lesions. In any case, surgery should be performed *early* in the presence of a deteriorating level of consciousness, although aggressive management of cerebellar hematomas is justified even in comatose patients. Ventricular enlargement is an important radiographic observation, since obstruction of cerebrospinal fluid flow may further aggravate ICP, and timely ventriculostomy may help control ICP. Because of problems with infection of ventricular shunts in the intensive care unit, ventriculostomy should not be carried out unless clearly indicated (i.e., this should not be a prophylactic procedure).[25] Unfortunately, because of the presence of blood in the cerebrospinal fluid, an internalized shunt is usually not feasible. We have used transcranial Doppler to help detect increasing ICP. As ICP increases, the diastolic velocity decreases, increasing the "pulsatility," which is a function of the difference between systolic and diastolic velocities. This may be an early clue to the need for ICP monitoring and surgical intervention.

The usual methods for controlling ICP, such as head elevation, mannitol or glycerol, and hyperventilation, as described in Chapter 4, are used in stroke patients.

SUBARACHNOID HEMORRHAGE

The treatment of aneurysmal subarachnoid hemorrhage has evolved substantially over the last 10 years. The main causes of morbidity and mortality, if a patient survives the acute hemorrhage, are recurrent hemorrhage and vasospasm. Recurrent hemorrhage can only be permanently prevented by definitive clipping of the offending aneurysm. Logically, the sooner this can be safely accomplished, the better the outcome. Recent evaluations of this problem have shown that early surgery may be advantageous, particularly in alert patients.[26] Therefore, patients with subarachnoid hemorrhage should have immediate arteriography and surgical clipping of the aneurysm within the first 3 days, if the aneurysm is easily accessible and the patient is alert. With more difficult-to-approach aneurysms, such as those on the anterior communicating artery or in the posterior fossa, and in patients with poor neurological status, surgery is generally deferred for approximately 2 weeks. Surgery after 3 to 4 days and before 10 days is usually not recommended, because this is the period of maximal vasospasm and morbidity and mortality are higher if surgery is carried out during this interval. While awaiting surgery, patients are usually put on anticonvulsants, stool softeners, and mild sedatives, and blood pressure is carefully controlled. Epsilon aminocaproic acid reduces the incidence of rebleeding, but seems to increase the complications of vasospasm.[27] This drug is still used by some neurologists and neurosurgeons to prevent fibrinolysis of the clot, which has formed around the aneurysm and stopped the subarachnoid bleeding. Patients who might benefit most from antifibrinolytics would be those with recurrent bleeding or with a particularly large aneurysm, in whom surgery is deferred for some reason and who are considered at relatively low risk for vasospasm.

The risk of vasospasm is directly related to the amount of subarachnoid bleeding. The etiology of vasospasm is poorly understood, but may be due to either neurogenic mechanisms or the interaction of the vessel wall with an as-yet-unidentified component of blood. Calcium antagonists, and in particular, nimodipine, have been proved effective for treating vasospasm.[28] Nimodipine reduces both mortality and morbidity from vasospasm, and calcium antagonists have now been shown to reduce vasospasm detected by arteriogram or transcranial Doppler. Nimodipine should be started in all patients as soon as subarachnoid hemorrhage is identified, and continued for 21 days. Other calcium antagonists, such as nicardipine, may also be effective and particularly useful when available in a parenteral formulation. Free radical scavengers are presently under evaluation for treatment of vasospasm. If vasospasm occurs after an aneurysm has been clipped, raising mean arterial blood pressure and volume expansion has been shown to reduce morbidity.[29] Volume expansion is best accomplished with a plasma substitute, albumin, or synthetic starch, and if aggressive volume expansion is carried out, Swan-Ganz catheterization should probably be used. Careful elevation of mean arterial blood pressure by 10 percent to 15 percent, using dopamine or dobutamine, may result in substantial improvement in patients with symptomatic vasospasm who have already had their aneurysm clipped.

ACUTE ISCHEMIC STROKE

The three strategies for treating acute cerebral infarction are antithrombotic therapy, reperfusion therapy, and neuronal protection.

Antithrombotic Therapy

Antithrombotic therapy with antiplatelet drugs or anticoagulants (heparin or warfarin) is commonly used but remains unproven therapy for acute strokes. Heparin is usually used to limit damage in those cases in which thrombosis of a large vessel is identified and the patient is neurologically unstable. Such conditions would include thrombosis of the carotid or basilar artery, sagittal sinus and other cerebral venous thrombosis, and dissection of the extracranial carotid or vertebral artery with secondary thrombus formation. Although most neurologists would use heparin in these clinical situations, the use of heparin has never been subjected to controlled prospective analysis. To avoid excessive anticoagulation, heparin is commonly used as a continuous intravenous infusion of 800 to 1,200 units/h with or without an initial bolus. Another situation in which heparin is used acutely is in patients considered at high risk for subsequent or recurrent stroke. This would include patients with TIAs and associated high-grade carotid stenosis, and patients with cardioembolic events secondary to underlying cardiac arrhythmia, mural thrombus, or valvular disease. In patients with TIAs and high-grade carotid stenosis, heparin is generally used only if the patient has had multiple TIAs despite antiplatelet therapy.

In patients with cardioembolic strokes, prospective studies have shown that heparin, followed by warfarin, substantially reduces the risk of recurrent embolization.[30] However, anticoagulation therapy should be withheld for 3 to 4 days after major cerebral infarction, even with a known cardioembolic source. This is because such infarcts often develop spontaneous hemorrhagic changes that can be aggravated by heparin therapy. A CT scan should be performed before initiating heparin or warfarin to be sure that no significant amount of hemorrhage is present. When anticoagulants are used, it is important to maintain careful control of blood pressure and avoid overanticoagulation (a bolus of heparin should not be given after cardioembolic stroke). Routine anticoagulation of all patients with acute ischemic stroke cannot be justified at the present time, although studies are now ongoing using low-molecular-weight heparin fractions to see if this type of anticoagulant therapy is effective and associated with acceptably low hemorrhagic risks.

Aspirin is commonly used if patients are not put on anticoagulants after acute ischemic stroke. Again, there are no prospective studies indicating that aspirin is effective in the acute stroke situation. Because long-term aspirin use has been shown to reduce the incidence of subsequent TIAs and strokes, patients should be started on platelet antiaggregant therapy at some time after their stroke to prevent recurrence. There is experimental evidence that platelet activation and production of arachidonic acid metabolites may aggravate post-ischemic injury. Therefore, aspirin started in the first few days after stroke may be beneficial, but this remains unproven.

Reperfusion Therapy

Reperfusion therapies are aimed at augmenting cerebral blood flow. Initially, vasodilators were tried, but they have generally been ineffective because blood vessels in ischemic regions are already maximally dilated. Other therapeutic efforts have included emergency thrombectomy. Although there have been some substantial successes with this type of operation, patients frequently developed severe cerebral edema, caused by reperfusion of necrotic tissue, and this outcome is difficult to predict prior to surgery. This aggressive type of reperfusion has largely been replaced by thrombolytic therapy.

Intra-arterial streptokinase and urokinase, as well as intravenous tissue plasminogen activator (tPA) and streptokinase, have been tried. The main concern with this form of therapy is that, as with thrombectomy, removal of an occluding thrombus or embolus and reperfusion of necrotic tissue may worsen the situation by causing cerebral edema and hemorrhage. The likelihood of hemorrhage could be increased even further by the systemic fibrinolytic effects of these drugs. For this reason, recent efforts have focused on early therapy, given before the development of tissue necrosis, and the use of intravenous tPA (which is associated with less systemic fibrinolysis), or intra-arterial infusion of urokinase proximal to the site of occlusion. A pilot study of tPA and one small controlled study from Japan have suggested that this therapy, in moderate doses, may be effective if started within the first few hours of stroke.[31, 32] Consequently, a randomized controlled study of tPA, stratified to include patients treated within 90 minutes and between 90 and 180 minutes of symptom onset, is presently underway. The 180-minute time window has been chosen because there appears to be progressively less benefit and more complications when thrombolytic treatment is started at intervals beyond 90 minutes. Furthermore, experimental studies in animals have shown that reperfusion must be started within 3 to 4 hours to result in reduced infarct size. Other trials of intravenous streptokinase are also underway.

If treatment is to be started within such a short interval, a minimum of diagnostic tests can be performed prior to therapy. In one ongoing evaluation of tPA, only a CT scan and routine blood studies are required to exclude cerebral hemorrhage, hypoglycemia, and underlying coagulopathy. In our center, we have enlisted the help of the emergency department staffs of eight hospitals as well as the city-wide paramedical system to enroll patients within these time windows. It is only possible to get treatment started within 90 minutes of acute stroke with extensive community education and close cooperation between paramedic and emergency department personnel. At most, we are able to treat one patient per month within 90 minutes and two within 180 minutes. Unless the time window can be pushed beyond the 90-minute period, it is unlikely that this form of therapy will benefit most stroke patients. Nevertheless, if thrombolytic therapy does prove to be effective, intensive community education efforts, as well as education of paramedic and emergency department staffs, may result in dramatic benefits in those patients reaching early therapy. Until present studies are completed, however, thrombolytic therapy should *not* be used outside of carefully designed and approved clinical research protocols. Even if blood pressure is controlled, there is no hemorrhage on CT, and treatment is begun early, cerebral hemorrhage and death from tPA therapy may still occur, so that until controlled trials show that the benefits substantially outweigh these risks, treatment outside clinical protocols should be avoided.

The final form of reperfusion therapy that has been commonly used is hemodilution. This is based on the theory that viscosity can be reduced by lowering red blood cell mass, and that decreased oxygen-carrying capacity occurring after hemodilution is more than compensated by increased cerebral blood flow resulting from reduction in viscosity. Unfortunately, several trials of isovolemic hemodilution using dextran plus phlebotomy have not shown any benefit in patients treated 12 to 24 hours after the onset of stroke.[33, 34] Whether this treatment would be more effective if started very early has not been evaluated, and deserves further study. However, it is clear that patients with acute cerebral ischemia do not tolerate hematocrits of much less than 35 percent or 36 percent. Relatively hypervolemic hemodilution adds the benefit of raising cardiac output by volume expansion. Unfortunately, in one study using this technique, increased cerebral edema occurred in patients treated with hypervolemic therapy.[35] Therefore, routine isovolemic or hypervolemic hemodilution cannot be recommended. However, in patients who are volume-depleted, it is important to replenish intravascular volume. In selected patients recognized early and without cerebral swelling, particularly if the hematocrit is greater than 45 percent, cautious hypervolemic therapy with 250 to 500 ml dextran or hydroxyethyl starch may be beneficial. If this treatment is undertaken, patients should have careful cardiovascular monitoring, probably with Swan-Ganz catheterization, to avoid precipitating congestive heart failure.

Neuronal Protection

The final strategy for treating acute cerebral infarction is neuronal protection. This is predicated on the contribution of disturbed calcium flux and calcium-activated enzyme systems to neuronal injury after ischemia and after other types of cerebral injury, such as hemorrhage, trauma, anoxia, and seizures. As a result of membrane depolarization and release of excitatory neurotransmitters, calcium enters neurons, consequently activating proteolytic enzymes and phospholipases. Many cellular perturbations ensue, including production of free radicals secondary to breakdown of membrane lipids. While the molecular biology of these postischemic events is still being unraveled, pharmacotherapy has focused on efforts to block calcium entry into neurons and prevent the production of free radicals. Experimental studies in animal stroke models have established a brief (several hours) window of opportunity to attenuate this cascade of events and consequent stroke severity.[36–39] The dihydropyridine calcium antagonists nimodipine and nicardipine dilate cerebral vessels and also block calcium entry into neurons.

To date, controlled trials of these drugs in stroke patients have not shown conclusive benefit, but treatment was started in most cases at least 24 hours after the onset of symptoms.[40] There is good evidence that those patients treated within 12 hours benefited.[41] A definitive trial of early treatment with a calcium antagonist remains to be carried out. These drugs have side effects, including hypotension and decreased cardiac output, so that the doses used have to be carefully titrated to prevent undesirable hemodynamic changes.

Antagonists of the excitatory neurotransmitter glutamate are more potent blockers of calcium entry into neurons, but may have behavioral side effects. These drugs are presently undergoing early clinical evaluation. Free radical scavengers (lazaroids) have shown dramatic results in experimental studies and are also under clinical investigation. Although conventional doses of glucocorticosteroids have not been shown to be effective in treating patients with acute stroke, it is possible that huge doses of these drugs may be beneficial as a result of their free radical scavenging activity. Other, even more experimental therapies presently in early stages of investigation include drugs that block the contribution of white blood cells to ischemic injury and platelet activating factor antagonists, which may prevent the consequences of arachidonic acid metabolism.

MIGRAINE

Severe complicated migraine headaches may mimic or cause acute strokes. Severe common migraine *without* associated neurological symptoms can be treated with intravenous infusions of dihydroergotamine (0.5 to 1.0 mg every 8 hours) along with an antiemetic (metoclopramide 10 mg every 8 hours).[42] Patients who have complicated migraine with associated neurological deficits should not be treated with such vasoconstrictors. At the present time, these patients should be treated with either a calcium antagonist such as verapamil (80 mg three times/day) or propranolol (40 to 60 mg three times/day). Sumatriptan, a newly developed serotonin antagonist, may prove to be particularly useful for treating all types of migraine headaches.[43]

REFERENCES

1. Silver FL, Norris JW, Lewis AJ, Hachinski VC: Early mortality following stroke: a prospective review. Stroke 15:492, 1984
2. Indredavik B, Bakke F, Solberg R et al: Benefit of a stroke unit: a randomized controlled trial. Stroke 22:1026, 1991
3. Mohr J, Sacco RL: Classification of ischemic strokes. p. 271. In Barnett HJM, Mohr JP, Stein BM, Yatsu FM (eds): Stroke: Pathophysiology, Diagnosis, and Management. 2nd Ed. Churchill Livingstone, New York, 1992
4. Levine SR, Brust JCM, Futrell N et al: A comparative study of the cerebrovascular complications of cocaine: alkaloidal versus hydrochloride—a review. Neurology 41:1173, 1991
5. Love B, Biller J: Stroke in the young. Stroke Clin Updates 4:13, 1990
6. Simon RP, Aminoff MJ, Greenberg DA: Clinical Neurology. Ch. 10. Appleton-Century-Crofts, East Norwalk, CT, 1989
7. Dusser A, Goutieres G, Aicardi H: Ischemic strokes in children. J Child Neurol 1:131, 1986
8. Barmada MA, Moosy J, Shuman RM: Cerebral infarcts with arterial occlusion in neonates. Ann Neurol 6:495, 1979
9. Levene M: Current Reviews in Paediatrics: Neonatal Neurology. Vol. 3. Churchill Livingstone, New York, 1987
10. Lanska MJ, Lanska DJ, Horwitz SJ, Aram DM: Presentation, clinical course, and outcome of childhood stroke. Pediatr Neurol 7:333, 1991
11. Roessmann U, Miller RT: Thrombosis of the middle cerebral artery associated with birth trauma. Neurology 30:889, 1980
12. Jackson AC, Boughner DR, Barnett HJM: Mitral valve prolapse and cerebral ischemic events in young patients. Neurology 34:784, 1984
13. Packer RJ, Rorke LB, Lange BJ et al: Cerebrovascular accidents in children with cancer. Pediatrics 76:194, 1985
14. Huttenlocher PR, Mohr JW, Johns L: Cerebral blood flow in sickle cell cerebrovascular disease. Pediatrics 73:615, 1984
15. Pavlakis SG, Phillips PC, DiMauro S et al: Mitochondrial myopathy, encephalopathy, lactic acidosis, and strokelike episodes: a distinctive clinical syndrome. Ann Neurol 16:481, 1984
16. Loes DJ, Smoker WRK, Biller J, Cornell SH: Nontraumatic lobar intracerebral hemorrhage: CT/angiographic correlation. AJNR 8:1027, 1987
17. Antiplatelet Trialists' Collaboration: Secondary prevention of vascular disease by prolonged antiplatelet treatment. Br Med J 296:320, 1988
18. Hass WK, Easton JD, Adams HP Jr et al: A randomized trial comparing ticlopidine hydrochloride with aspirin for the prevention of stroke in high risk patients. N Engl J Med 321:501, 1989
19. Grotta JC, Norris JW, Kamm B, TASS Baseline and Angiographic Data Sub-Group: Prevention of stroke with ticlopidine: who benefits most? Neurology 42:111, 1992
20. North American Symptomatic Carotid Endarterectomy Trial Collaborators: Beneficial effect of carotid endarterectomy in symptomatic patients with high-grade carotid stenosis. N Engl J Med 325:445, 1991
21. Grotta JC, Pettigrew LC, Allen S et al: Baseline hemodynamic state and response to hemodilution in patients with acute cerebral ischemia. Stroke 16:790, 1985
22. Ameriso SF, Wong VLY, Quismorio FP Jr, Fisher M: Immunohematologic characteristics of infection-associated cerebral infarction. Stroke 22:1004, 1991
23. Kushner M, Nencini P, Reivich M, et al: Relationship of hyperglycemia early in

ischemic brain infarction to cerebral anatomy, metabolism, and clinical outcome. Ann Neurol 28:129, 1990

24. Broderick JP, Brott TG, Tomsick T et al: Ultra-early evaluation of intracerebral hemorrhage. J Neurosurg 72:195, 1990

25. Heros RC: Acute hydrocephalus after subarachnoid hemorrhage. Stroke 20:715, 1989

26. Kassel NF, Torner JC, Jane JA et al: The International Cooperative Study on the Timing of Aneurysm Surgery—part 2: surgical results. J Neurosurg 73:37, 1990

27. Vermeulen M, Lindsay KW, Murray GD et al: Antifibrinolytic treatment in subarachnoid hemorrhage. N Engl J Med 311:432, 1984

28. Pickard JD, Murray GD, Illingworth R et al: Effect of oral nimodipine on cerebral infarction and outcome after subarachnoid hemorrhage: British Aneurysm Nimodipine Trial. Br Med J 298:636, 1989

29. Awad IA, Carter LP, Spetzler RF et al: Clinical vasospasm after subarachnoid hemorrhage: response to hypervolemic hemodilution and arterial hypertension. Stroke 18:365, 1987

30. Cerebral Embolism Task Force: Cardiogenic brain embolism. Arch Neurol 46:727, 1989

31. Brott T, Haley C, Levy D et al: Safety and potential efficacy of tissue plasminogen activator (tPA) for stroke. Stroke 21:181, 1990

32. Mori E, Yoneda Y, Ohksawa S et al: Double-blind, placebo-controlled trial of recombinant tissue plasminogen activator (rt-PA) in acute carotid stroke. Neurology 41(suppl. 1):347, 1991

33. Scandinavian Stroke Study Group: Multicenter trial of hemodilution in acute ischemic stroke: results in the total patient population. Stroke 18:691, 1987

34. Italian Acute Stroke Study Group: Haemodilution in acute stroke: results of the Italian Haemodilution Trial. Lancet 1:318, 1988

35. Hemodilution in Stroke Study Group: Hypervolemic hemodilution treatment of acute stroke: results of a randomized multicenter trial using pentastarch. Stroke 20:317, 1989

36. Hass WK: Beyond cerebral blood flow, metabolism and ischemic thresholds: an examination of the role of calcium in the initiation of cerebral infarction. In Meyer JS, Lechner H, Reivich M et al (eds): Cerebral Vascular Disease 3: Proceedings of the 10th International Salzburg Conference, September 24–27. Excerpta Medica, Amsterdam, 1981

37. Raichle ME: The pathophysiology of brain ischemia. Ann Neurol 13:2, 1983

38. Steen PA, Newberg IA, Milde JH, Michenfelder JD: Nimodipine improves cerebral blood flow and neurologic recovery after complete cerebral ischemia in the dog. J Cereb Blood Flow Metab 3:38, 1983

39. Picone CM, Grotta JC, Earls J et al: Immunohistochemical determination of calcium-calmodulin binding predicts neuronal damage after global ischemia. J Cereb Blood Flow Metab 9:805, 1989

40. Mohr JP, Dilanni M, Muschett JL et al: Nimodipine in acute ischemic stroke. Ann Neurol 26:124, 1989

41. Rosenbaum DM, Zambramski J, Frey J et al: Early treatment of ischemic stroke with a calcium antagonist. Stroke 22:437, 1991

42. Raskin NH: Repetitive intravenous dihydroergotamine as a therapy for intractable migraine. Neurology 36:995, 1986

43. Subcutaneous Sumatriptan International Study Group: Treatment of migraine attacks with sumatriptan. N Engl J Med 325:316, 1991

3

Diagnosis and Treatment of Head Injury

Russ P. Nockels
Lawrence H. Pitts

Head injury remains a leading cause of death and disability in young adults. Nearly half of all traumatic deaths are the result of head injury, with the mechanism bearing a relationship to local factors: vehicular trauma predominates in high-traffic areas, while assault is more common in socioeconomically depressed regions. Head injured patients are three times more likely to be male, and are typically in their second or third decade of life.

While little can be done about the impact damage to the brain, emphasis should be placed on early clinical evaluation, recognition of neurological course, and prevention of so-called *secondary* insults, which negatively impact upon survival and subsequent function. Recognition of the importance of these events, such as hypoxemia, hypotension, and intracranial hypertension, has led to the institution of fundamental guidelines for diagnosis and management. While optimal treatment of head injury remains elusive, the impact of these guidelines is enormous when considering the devastating consequences of missed diagnosis and improper therapy.

The concept that brain injury can *evolve* carries with it a weighty responsibility. It is becoming increasingly clear that, immediately after injury, a state of enhanced vulnerability is produced for many important regions of the brain. Our understanding of the basic mechanisms underlying permanent neuronal damage has helped to define important clinical events during this state of vulnerability. For instance, it is quite clear that the brain itself has minimal reserves of energy substrate when faced with compromise of its nutrients. The cerebral cortex and hippocampus are particularly sensitive in the acute post-traumatic state to systemic events that are otherwise not deleterious to the uninjured brain, such as moderate hypoxemia. In addition, the restorative capacity of the brain is severely limited in the mature central nervous system. Taken together, these are compelling arguments for the earliest possible recognition of head injury and immediate intervention to maintain normal cerebral blood flow, oxygenation, and intracranial pressure following trauma.

PATHOLOGY

The clinically relevant forms of damage occurring after head injury are a continuum of insults, generally thought to begin with axonal shearing. As a consequence of rapid acceleration and deceleration, the structural integrity of the axons is disrupted, leading to the formation of axonal retraction bulbs. These microscopic events may be found, diffusely, throughout the white matter of the cerebral hemispheres, or (less commonly) focally, within the corpus callosum or rostral brain stem. The term *diffuse axonal injury* is used to describe a clinical correlate to this phenomenon. Brain swelling secondary to loss of homeostatic protective mechanisms may follow, both from extra and intracellular increases in water and ionic content, as well as abnormal vasodilatation. The blood brain barrier becomes dysfunctional in broad cerebral territories during this time. Areas of direct contact between brain and bone (such as the frontal and temporal poles, which contact the skull base) may progress into contusions. These are heralded by extravasation of blood and displacement of the surrounding brain. Pial vessel disruption or laceration of bridging vessels between the brain and dural sinuses may cause hemorrhage into the subdural space. Vessels nourishing the skull and dura, particularly the middle meningeal artery, may become lacerated, especially if a skull fracture is present, and cause hemorrhage within the epidural space.

If the damage remains confined, neurological function specific to that brain region will be focally impaired. If the sum total of these events, however, leads to mass effect sufficient to cause brain distortion and brain stem compression, profound deficits in consciousness may occur. Eventually, as vital brain stem areas fail, death occurs. Understanding the sequence of these events leads to a greater understanding that some patients *can* perish as the result of correctable factors, such as increased intracranial pressure and/or the presence of a surgically removable hematoma. The basis for a general approach to head injury, therefore, is to recognize and rapidly treat these patients.

GENERAL APPROACH

The initial evaluation of head injury begins outside the central nervous system. As in any patient sustaining significant trauma, the first focus should be on the adequacy of the airway and maintenance of near-normal hemodynamics. Complicating factors are common, as hypoxemia ($PO_2 < 60$ mm Hg) accompanies up to 65 percent of head injuries,[1] while hypotension is present in 16 to 31 percent.[2,3] Stabilization of any major systemic injury causing hypotension or hypoxemia is imperative in minimizing secondary brain injury. In addition, it is a prerequisite to determining the degree of neurological impairment, as these systemic factors can mask neurological deficit and—of similar importance—subsequent deterioration. Post-traumatic seizures are treated under the same guidelines as status epilepticus. When necessary, placement of an endotracheal tube should follow, under axial cervical traction to avoid dislocation of an occultly injured spine. While the optimal resuscitative fluid has not been defined, it is generally accepted that colloid contributes less to cerebral edema than crystalloids during acute periods of cerebral insult. In patients with isolated head injury, the standard trauma administration of several liters of intravenous volume should obviously be avoided.

Following resuscitation, the baseline neurological exam should be determined. This critical stage of the evaluation allows two simple questions to be answered. First, are any focal signs present? Residual post-traumatic function can be just as important to management as deficit. For example, a post-traumatic hemiplegia may indicate either the discrete loss of cerebral function underlying a depressed skull fracture, profound brain stem compression accompanying a herniation syndrome, or a Brown-Séquard spinal cord injury. Taken in combination with the presence or absence of other deficits (such as coma and a contralateral pupillary abnormality indicative of herniation), focal signs can direct acute investigations and management.

Second, what is the patient's course—one of recovery, deterioration, or a plateau phase? One often gains very useful insight into the neurological course through observations made at the scene by witnesses or emergency personnel. The potential factor of intoxicating substances often confounds the acute neurological evaluation. Intoxicated patients who *appear* to be neurologically impaired characteristically recover given time; those with actual mass lesions almost inevitably deteriorate, underscoring the importance of vigilance in all cases.

It is obviously vital to have a reliable measure of injury to serve as a basis of comparison for future exams. The Glasgow coma scale (GCS) (Table 3-1) was developed as a semiquantitative method of measuring head injury, taking into account three reliable indicators of post-traumatic dysfunction (eye opening, language capability, and movement).[4] The exam is invalid in children and intoxicated patients, or when concomitant orbital or spinal cord injury is present. Patients with a GCS score of less than 8 are usually defined as severe, while moderate and mild injuries have GCS scores of 9 to 12 and 13 to 15, respectively. Following determination of the GCS score, the cranial nerves should be inspected sequentially. It is imperative that extraocular movements never be checked with a Doll's eye maneuver until the cervical spine is cleared on both radiographic and clinical grounds. Pupillary response to light and extremity response to painful stimuli (such as a trapezius pinch) are useful in identifying localized deficits caused by uncal or transtentorial herniation.

It is logical to assume intracranial hypertension in any patient with a GCS score of less than 8. Focal findings, particularly a defective ipsilateral pupillary response to light stimulus and frank posturing, indicate the presence of an expanding intracranial mass. A basic diagnostic tenet is that an ipsilateral pupillary defect is a more reliable indicator of lesion side than a contralateral hemiplegia, since, in up to 25 percent of cases, the motor deficit is ipsilateral (Kernohan's notch phenomenon). Immediate attempts to lower intracranial pressure, including hyperventilation to a PCO_2 of 30 mmHg and the adminis-

Table 3-1. GLASGOW COMA SCALE

Eye Opening:		
Spontaneous		4
To speech		3
To pain		2
Nothing		1
Best *Motor* Response:		
Obeys		6
Localizes		5
Withdraws		4
Abnormal flexion		3
Extensor response		2
Flaccid		1
Best *Verbal* Response:		
Oriented		5
Confused conversation		4
Inappropriate words		3
Incomprehensible sounds		2
Nothing		1
Total (*E* + *M* + *V*)		3–15

(From Teasdale and Jennett,[4] with permission.)

tration of intravenous 5 percent mannitol (1.5 g/kg), are mandatory under these circumstances. In most institutions, a computed tomography (CT) scan of the brain is obtained to confirm or refute the suspicion of mass lesion. In treating patients with mechanisms of injury much more likely to produce intracranial hematomas, particularly in younger patients without vehicular trauma, the patient may be taken immediately to the operating room for burr-hole exploration and evacuation of any significant lesion through craniotomy.[5] CT scan may also be necessary in awake patients if a depressed skull fracture is suspected, or a cerebrospinal fluid leak is present.

The majority of patients evaluated for head injury have sustained a mild or moderate injury (GCS scores of 13 to 15 or 8 to 12, respectively). While the mortality in these patients is quite low, a period of intensive observation is necessary to determine the evolution, if any, of neurological symptoms. For this reason, any post-traumatic patient with an altered level of consciousness is admitted to the hospital overnight for frequent observation. Patients with GCS scores of 15 may be discharged if an appropriate guardian is available. Intracranial pressure-reducing measures are introduced only if deterioration takes place. While routine CT scanning of this population is often reassuring, its cost-effectiveness is controversial, and certainly should not substitute for frequent careful observation.[6]

The value of routine and standardized evaluation of all patients with any diminution in level of consciousness after head injury is paramount. The state of spontaneous arousal and the degree of response to both verbal and tactile stimuli are inherent features of the GCS evaluation, and are best appreciated by the same examiner in a repetitive fashion. Any deterioration requires immediate assessment with CT scan or, if severe enough, support and treatment for increased intracranial pressure. For this reason, it is best not to paralyze and intubate patients with mild or moderate injury (GCS scores of 13 to 15 and 9 to 12, respectively), as this invariably leads to a loss of the ability to assess neurological course.

Often the first irrefutable evidence of a head injury is the presence of a scalp laceration. Following the neurological examination, an assessment of the scalp and skull is required to determine if large lacerations overlay compound skull fractures, and whether oto- or rhinorrhea is present. Obvious scalp lacerations greater than a fingerbreadth in width are carefully probed with a sterile, gloved finger to determine the presence or absence of an underlying skull fracture. A *step off*, or palpable bony shelf, is assumed to represent a depressed fracture, and requires CT evaluation. Due to the risk of infection, severe comminuted fractures require operative exploration, with débridement of any underlying brain contamination and repair of the dural laceration.[7,8] Closed skull vault fractures, the benchmark of head injury, are of little significance in awake patients if they are not depressed, save that they indicate a severe blow. Basal skull fractures are often heralded by cutaneous manifestations or, less commonly, a focal neurological deficit. Again, CT scan will often define the fracture. Some controversy exists regarding elevation of depressed fractures where infection is not a concern.[8]

The incidence of cerebrospinal fluid leak in patients with closed head injury is 2 to 6 percent.[8-11] Racoon and Battle signs are two common superficial manifestations of a basal skull defect, and should prompt concern about a cerebrospinal fluid oto- or rhinorrhea. The clinical presentation depends on the site of the bony defect. In the case of anterior cranial trauma and disruption of the cribiform plate, drainage will occur either through the nares or postnasal space. If the fracture involves the petromastoid region, cerebrospinal fluid will leak through the middle ear, unless the tympanic membrane is intact in which case it may be diverted through the eustachian tube and into the oropharynx. In such cases, patients may note a dripping sensation or salty taste in the throat. It is our practice to manage these patients with bedrest, head elevation, and moderate fluid restriction. The outlook is very good for this component of the injury. Approximately 85 percent of post-traumatic rhinorrhea and nearly all cases of otorrhea resolve within the first week of conservative measures.[8-11] Persistent cerebrospinal fluid leaks may require surgical exploration and repair of the dural defect to prevent meningitis.

Cranial nerves are susceptible to injury when they traverse a skull fracture. The facial nerve is the most commonly injured cranial nerve, complicating 0.3 to 5 percent of all head injuries, and 25 percent of all fractures involving the petromastoid region.[12,13] The nerve can be lacerated across the fractured bony edge on impact, or become compressed over time by swelling within the narrow fallopian canal. One should make every effort to determine the timing and degree of facial nerve dysfunction, as the prognosis for spontaneous recovery depends on whether the deficit was immediate or delayed, complete or partial. Recovery occurs in nearly 100 percent of delayed partial injuries, in contrast to only 50 percent of immediate complete facial palsies.[12,13] The optic nerve is also commonly injured, a situation that obviously complicates pupillary assessment due to an afferent defect. Interestingly, axonal injuries within the optic nerve are very similar to those seen in the cerebral white matter in diffuse axonal injury.[14]

INTRACRANIAL HEMATOMAS

The progression of post-traumatic patients into coma, with the development of pupillary hyporeactivity and abnormal posturing, is assumed to be due to mass lesions. All efforts should, again, be directed toward rapid diagnosis and treatment. The most common finding is the combination of intracerebral contusion and subdural hematoma, followed by the finding of epidural or subdural hematomas alone.[15] Even under optimal management, the outcomes for these types of lesions are quite different.

Epidural hematomas are often heralded by an initial post-traumatic period of near-normal function, followed several hours later by coma and hemiplegia. This so-called "lucid" interval, however, is a nonspecific indicator of lesion type, and is an obvious indication that the impact injury to the brain was relatively minor. Often there is a history of brief loss of consciousness at the time of injury as well. The slow development of these symptoms is thought to be due to the stubbornness of the dura in adhering to the inner table of the calvarium as the hematoma collects. This adherence is a function of age, explaining why epidural hematoma is rare in patients over 60 years of age. Since the skull has absorbed a great deal of the impact force, the brain is often relatively spared. This further explains why the mortality rate for treated epidural hematomas in this country is approaching 5 percent.[16,17] Untreated (often unrecognized) epidural hematoma carries a mortality rate of 40 to 100 percent.

Subdural hematomas carry much more dramatic consequences. Even with treatment, mortality rates range from 42 to 90 percent.[18–20] The most important factor affecting outcome is the preoperative neurological status, with mortality rates of greater than 75 percent in patients with GCS scores of 3 to 5.[21] As with all other forms of head injury, age is also a decisive factor, with mortality rates of 19 percent for patients less than 40 years of age, and 62 percent in those over that age.[20]

Intracerebral hematomas range in significance from incidentally discovered contusions to rapidly expanding mass lesions requiring operative removal. CT scan demonstrates such lesions in 6 to 30 percent of all head-injured patients.[15] Hemorrhage into an area of contusion can occur in a delayed fashion and is thought to be a cause of late deterioration. Such events, occurring within days to weeks of the injury, are termed *delayed traumatic intracerebral hematomas.*[22] As these lesions occupy increasing intracranial space, they may produce mass effect, prompting their diagnosis through clinical deterioration. Removal of these contusions is usually reserved for patients with progressive symptoms or uncontrollable intracranial pressure.[23] The relatively high mortality rates in these patients (between 25 to 60 percent in large series[23–25] is related to the severity of the injury producing the hematoma as well as the hematoma itself.

PENETRATING TRAUMA

Civilian gunshot wounds to the head represent the most common form of penetrating head injury, as well as the most lethal, and many patients do not survive to be evaluated by a neurosurgeon. Such penetrating wounds cause not only direct mechanical trauma to the brain, but are commonly associated with intracerebral and extracerebral hematomas. The passage of a high energy shock wave can cause massive destruction, which accounts for the high mortality. Yet, some of these patients do survive to lead productive lives, therefore, the major acute issue is who should or should not be aggressively treated.[26]

In general, patients presenting in coma with abnormal motor posturing and bilateral cerebral injury (as indicated by plain film or CT scan) do not survive, regardless of treatment.[27-29] Those with focal neurological deficit or with primarily mass lesions may benefit from operative care. In these patients, consideration must also be given to débridement of entrance or exit wounds to prevent infection.

FUTURE THERAPY

As the focus of head injury care shifts from patient survival to survivor function, novel therapies can be tested for clinical benefit. These treatments should target post-traumatic alterations in the brain's endogenous biochemistry, such as the production and release of autodestructive factors and the overstimulation of membrane receptors. For example: the endocrinologic activities of methylprednisolone were once thought necessary to reduce post-traumatic tissue damage. However, experimental dose-response studies suggest that methylprednisolone's *biochemical* actions, such as the inhibition of free radical generated lipid peroxidation may be of sole importance.[30] This has led to the development of man-made steroids that are potent inhibitors of lipid peroxidation yet have no glucocorticoid activity and, theoretically, fewer side effects.[31,32] One such compound, U74006F, or Tirilazad (Upjohn), is now undergoing a multicenter head and spinal cord injury trial.

Blockade of the overexcitation of excitatory amino acid and opiate receptors has had promising effects on head injured animals, and may lead to compounds safe and effective for human use.[33,34] These compounds hold particular promise because their anatomic sites of action are the hippocampus and cerebral cortex.

Since even normal cell metabolism during periods of nutrient deprivation can lead to cell death, some investigators are focusing on reducing metabolic rate, either through barbiturate therapy or hypothermia. The induction of "pentobarbital coma" for head injury has been limited to severely injured patients with uncontrolled intracranial hypertension. Negative interaction between barbiturate treatment and cardiopulmonary systems has curtailed its use to a small subset of patients, but this type of treatment should be considered in refractory patients following exhaustive conservative measures to reduce intracranial pressure. Since little alternative exists in controlling intracranial pressure in patients without mass lesions, some centers have begun treating patients with barbiturates earlier in their course.[35] Efforts to define therapeutic parameters of hypothermia have demonstrated a significant disparity between brain and systemic temperature in head-injured patients. While experimental evidence for the safety of hypothermia increases, the systemic consequences of both these treatments may limit their clinical use.[36]

CONCLUSION

The single most important defense against avoidable and permanent neurological dysfunction in the head-injured patient is the informed observer. Utilizing these guidelines, with complementary knowledge of the processes contributing to avoidable deficits, the rational treatment of these patients can have long lasting effects.

REFERENCES

1. Frost EAM, Arancibia CU, Schulman K: Pulmonary shunt as a prognosticator in head injury. J Neurosurg 50:768, 1979
2. Eisenberg HM, Cayard C, Papanicolaou A et al: The effect of three potentially preventable complications on outcome after severe closed head injury. p. 549. In Ishii S, Nagai H, Brock M (eds): Intracranial Pressure Vol. 5. Springer-Verlag, Tokyo, 1983
3. Miller JD, Sweet RC, Narayan RK et al: Early insults to the injured brain. JAMA 240:439, 1978
4. Teasdale G, Jennett B: Assessment of coma and impaired consciousness—a practical scale. Lancet 2:81, 1974
5. Andrews BT, Pitts LH, Lovely MP et al: Is computed tomography scanning necessary in patients with transtentorial herniation? Results of immediate surgical exploration without computed tomography in 100 patients. Neurosurgery 19:408, 1986
6. Dacey RG, Alves, WM, Rimel RW: Neurosurgical complications after apparently mild head injury. J Neurosurg 65:203, 1986
7. Cooper PR: Skull Fracture and Traumatic Cerebrospinal Fluid Fistulas. p. 89. In Cooper PR (ed): Head Injury. Williams & Wilkins, Baltimore, 1987
8. Van den Heever HJ, Van der Merwe DJ: Management of depressed skull fractures: selective conservative management of nonmissile injuries. J Neurosurg 71:186, 1989
9. Laun A: Traumatic cerebrospinal fluid fistulas in the anterior and middle cranial fossae. Acta Neurochir (Wien) 60:215, 1982
10. Leech PJ, Paterson A: Conservative and operative management for cerebrospinal fluid leakage after closed head injury. Lancet 1:1013, 1973
11. Lewin W: CSF rhinorrhea in nonmissile head injuries. Clin Neurosurg 12:237, 1966
12. Curtin JM: Fractures of the skull and intratemporal lesions affecting the facial nerve. Adv Otorhinolaryngol 22:202, 1977
13. Turner JWA: Facial palsy in closed head injuries. Lancet 2:756, 1944
14. Rovit RL, Murali R: Injuries of the cranial nerves. p. 141. In Cooper PR (ed): Head Injury. Williams & Wilkins, Baltimore, 1987
15. Jennett B, Teasdale G (eds): Management of head injuries. FA Davis, Philadelphia, 1981

16. Baykaner K, Alp H, Cerviker N et al: Observation of 95 patients with extradural hematoma and review of the literature. Surg Neurol 30:399, 1988

17. Bricolo AP, Pasut LM: Extradural hematoma: toward zero mortality. Neurosurgery 14:8, 1984

18. Gennarelli TA, Thibault LE: Biomechanics of acute subdural hematoma. J Trauma 22:680, 1982

19. Seelig JM, Becker DP, Miller JD et al: Traumatic acute subdural hematoma. Major morbidity reduction in comatose patients treated within four hours. N Engl J Med 304:1511, 1981

20. Stone JL, Rifai MHS, Sugar O et al: Acute subdural hematoma: progress in definition, clinical pathology, and therapy. Surg Neurol 19:216, 1983

21. Gennarelli TA, Spielman GM, Langfitt TW et al: Influence of the type of intracranial lesion on outcome from severe head injury. J Neurosurg 56:26, 1982

22. Fukamachi A, Nagaseki Y, Kohno K et al: The incidence and developmental process of delayed traumatic intracerebral hematomas. Acta Neurochir (Wein) 74:35, 1985

23. Bullock R, Golek J, Blake G: Traumatic intracerebral hematoma: which patients should undergo surgical evaluation? CT scan features and ICP monitoring as a basis for decision making. Surg Neurol 32:181, 1989

24. Piepmeier J, Wagner FC: Delayed post-traumatic intracerebral hematomas. J Trauma 22:455, 1982

25. Teasdale G, Golbraith S: Acute traumatic intracranial hematomas. p. 252. In Krayenbuhl H, Maspes PE, Sweet WH (eds): Progress in Neurological Surgery. S Karger, Basel, 1980

26. Kaufman HH, Makela ME, Lee KF et al: Gunshot wounds to the head: a perspective. Neurosurgery 18:689, 1986

27. Kaufman HH, Loyala WP, Makela ME et al: Civilian gunshot wounds: the limits of salvageability. Acta Neurochir (Wein) 67:115, 1983

28. Nagib MG, Rockswold GL, Sherman RS et al: Civilian gunshot wounds to the brain. Neurosurgery 18:533, 1986

29. Clark WC, Muhlbauer MS, Watridge CB et al: Analysis of 76 civilian craniocerebral gunshot wounds. J Neurosurg 65:9, 1986

30. Hall ED, Braughler JM: The role of oxygen radical induced lipid peroxidation in acute central nervous system trauma. p. 92. In Halliwell B (ed): Oxygen Radicals and Tissue Injury. Federation of American Societies for Experimental Biology, Bethesda, 1988

31. Hall ED, Yonkers, PA, McCall UM et al: Effects of the 21-aminosteroid U74006F on experimental head injury in mice. J Neurosurg 68:456, 1988

32. Dimlich RVW, Tornheim PA, Kindel RM, Hall ED et al: Effects of a 21-aminosteroid (U74006F) on cerebral metabolites and edema after severe experimental head trauma. In Long D (ed): Advances in Neurology. Raven Press, New York, 1990

33. Albers GW, Goldberg MP, Choi DW: N-methyl-D-aspartate antagonists: ready for clinical trial in brain ischemia? Ann Neurol 25:398, 1989

34. Faden AI, Demediuk P, Panter SS et al: The role of excitatory amino acids and NMDA receptors in traumatic brain injury. Science 244:798, 1989

35. Eisenberg H, Frankowski RF, Contant C et al: High-dose barbiturate control of elevated intracranial pressure in patients with severe head injury. J Neurosurg 69:15, 1988

36. Hoff JT: Cerebral protection. J Neurosurg 65:579, 1986

4

Intracranial Pressure Monitoring and Cerebral Resuscitation

Michael A. Williams
Daniel F. Hanley

INTRACRANIAL PRESSURE AND
CEREBRAL MONITORING

Safe and effective care of patients with critical neurological compromise depends on rapid intervention and physiologic monitoring so that the outcome of interventions may be modified. Traditional neurological practice relies on changes in the patient's neurological examination as the primary physiologic monitoring technique. The neurological examination is a sensitive test that may reveal changing function in virtually every part of the nervous system when properly performed with an awake, cooperative patient. However, the sensitivity declines in patients with altered levels of consciousness and coma, in whom only a limited number of reflex responses may be elicited for monitoring purposes. In such patients, critical changes in intracranial pressure (ICP), cerebral blood flow (CBF), neurotransmission, and cortical electrical activity may occur with minimal or no changes in the external appearance of the patient. The ability to monitor and modify physiologic variables has proved of benefit in rendering care and has improved the neurological outcome in a number of processes, including intracranial hypertension,[1,2] status epilepticus,[3–5] and delayed vasospasm associated with subarachnoid hemorrhage.[6,7]

This chapter describes contemporary brain monitoring techniques and the approaches to cerebral resuscitation that may be undertaken with their use.

INTRACRANIAL PRESSURE MONITORING

The importance of ICP in cerebral injury was first demonstrated by Guillaume and Janny,[8] and then by Lundberg.[9] ICP monitoring has been used in conjunction with improved outcome of closed head injury,[1,10] acute hydrocephalus, and Reye syndrome.[11] Further work has shown that cerebral perfusion pressure (CPP) is as important as ICP, if not more so.[12,13] CPP is operationally defined as CPP = MABP − ICP (or JVP), where MABP is mean arterial blood pressure and JVP is jugular venous pressure; the greater of ICP or JVP is used. Therefore, standard practice in the care of patients with intracranial hypertension is to monitor both ICP and arterial blood pressure to permit continuous CPP assessment. Several good reviews of the physiology of ICP and CPP are available.[14,15]

Currently, available ICP monitoring techniques are divided between fluid-coupled systems with external transducers, such as intraventricular catheters (IVC) and subarachnoid bolts (SA bolt), and fiber optic systems, which use a miniature pressure transducer within a catheter that may be inserted in the lateral ventricle, brain parenchyma, subarachnoid space, or epidural space.

Fluid-coupled Systems

Fluid-coupled systems with external transducers can be calibrated accurately, reproducibly, and in conjunction with arterial blood pressure monitoring. The accuracy of the transduced pressure depends on the anatomic location of the communication between the fluid column and the intracranial space. Traditionally, the most accurate and reliable pressure waveforms are obtained through IVCs, which measure pressure from the lateral ventricle deep within the brain. The IVC waveform is not susceptible to error or damping unless there is air or a thick blood clot within the ventricle or tubing or brain edema sufficient to collapse the ventricles against the catheter. The IVC is particularly useful when the lateral ventricles are enlarged because it may be used to drain cerebrospinal fluid (CSF), and thus functions as both a monitor and a treatment for intracranial hypertension. The IVC is also used in normal-sized ventricles, but it is difficult to insert into collapsed ventricles, as would be found with diffuse cerebral edema. In such a situation, an SA bolt or fiber optic system are more appropriate to use.

The IVC is inserted in the intensive care unit (ICU), the emergency department, or the operating room. The most common insertion site is over the posterior frontal lobe, preferably in the nondominant hemisphere. A 3- to 4-cm skin incision and burr hole are made 2 cm lateral to the sagittal suture and 2 cm anterior to the coronal suture. The catheter is then passed to a depth of 6 to 8 cm, aiming for the contralateral medial canthus while staying in the interauricular plane. Once CSF is encountered, the catheter is connected to pressure tubing and an external drainage system via a three-way stopcock. The pressure transducer is kept at the level of the external acoustic meatus for calibration and monitoring.

The main risks of IVCs are infection and complications of insertion. The infection rate varies from 0 percent to 27 percent.[16–18] The risk of IVC-associated meningitis or ventriculitis appears to be related to the duration of catheter insertion. Mayhall et al[17] found the risk of infection increased from 9 percent on day 5 to 21 percent on day 8 and to 42 percent on day 11. Others, however, have reported no association of infection with catheter duration.[16,18] Mayhall and colleagues[17] found additional risk factors for infection were irrigation of the drainage system and intraventricular blood, but insertion of the IVC in the ICU posed no additional risk of infection compared with insertion in the operating room. Because of the high infection risk, our practice is to administer prophylactic antibiotics as long as the IVC is in place. The insertion technique is blind, and it is possible to cause a parenchymal hemorrhage, which probably occurs when a pial vessel is stretched or torn. Rarely, injury of vital structures such as the thalamus, hypothalamus, or midbrain occurs if the IVC is passed too deep.

Subarachnoid Bolt

The SA bolt is indicated for ICP monitoring when CSF drainage is neither feasible nor desired. The skull insertion site is similar to the IVC, except that there is more freedom to place the SA bolt at different sites because the brain parenchyma is not punctured. Skull stability, the side of cerebral pathology, and evidence of pre-existing skin disease are the most important criteria for site selection. After a burr hole is made, the hollow, self-tapping bolt is inserted into the skull, and the dura at the base of the bolt is perforated with a spinal needle to allow subarachnoid CSF to fill the bolt. Saline-filled pressure tubing is then connected to establish communication to the pressure monitoring system. The SA bolt usually provides a reliable ICP waveform and pressure reading, but it is susceptible to error if the dural perforations become plugged with blood or debris or if brain swelling obliterates communication with CSF. Debris may be flushed from the bolt with 0.5 ml nonbacteriostatic saline solution. In particular, the SA bolt tends to underestimate ICP when it is elevated.[19] Because the SA bolt measures the local ICP at the surface of the hemisphere, it may be inaccurate if there is a pressure differential between the left and right supratentorial compartments.[20] The existence of compartmental pressure differences is debatable, however, and some studies have shown no difference in ICP measured simultaneously ipsilateral and contralateral to a hemispheric lesion.[21] Johnston and Rowan[22] demonstrated gradients between the supratentorial and infratentorial compartments. The SA bolt is only a monitoring instrument; CSF cannot be withdrawn from it. The infection risk is extremely low, probably because the brain and ventricles are not penetrated. In our ICU, we have seen one local wound infection and no central nervous system infections associated with SA bolts in 8 years (unpublished data). We do not administer prophylactic antibiotics for SA bolts.

Fiber Optic Systems with Miniature Transducers

Current ICP monitors with implantable miniature transducers are coupled with fiber optic cables. A transducer is incorporated into the end of a soft tube that may be solid, or may be hollow and function like an IVC. The fiber optic system operates by projecting light through an optic fiber to a tiny, displaceable mirror in the catheter tip.[23] The amount of light reflected to a collecting optic fiber depends on the displacement of the mirror, which, in turn, is a function of ICP. As such, this is a photometric transduction system. Such transducers may be inserted in the lateral ventricle, the brain parenchyma, the subarachnoid space, or the epidural space. Their greatest advantage is that they do not require fluid coupling for pressure transduction, which avoids the problems of waveform damping and artifacts from poor coupling and also allows for the wide choice of insertion sites. A major disadvantage is that the transducer cannot be calibrated to zero once it has been inserted. Its accuracy, as compared with the IVC, has been shown in the subdural space, the brain parenchyma, and the ventricles,[24-26] although a recent report showed that parenchymal fiber optic pressures exceeded IVC pressures by a mean of 9.2 mmHg and, in some instances, by as much as 40 mmHg.[27] The fiber optic device has sufficient baseline drift after 5 days use (± 6 mmHg) to cause significant inaccuracy and the need for replacement.[24] In early versions, the optic fibers were inflexible and broke easily, but this is less of a problem with current models. The fiber optic system is not directly compatible with many ICU bedside monitoring and patient data management systems and must be connected to a separate module to be used, which may increase the cost of ICP monitoring. The risk of infection with these devices would be expected to depend on the insertion site, and should be similar to the risk for IVCs or SA bolts.

TRANSCRANIAL DOPPLER SONOGRAPHY

Transcranial Doppler sonography (TCD) was developed and first reported by Aaslid et al in 1982.[28] The technique involves transmitting low-energy ultrasonic pulses through the skull either at its thinnest point (the temporal bone) or through foramina, such as the superior orbital fissure or the foramen magnum. The sound waves are reflected by flowing blood and returned to the TCD receiver. Changes in the frequency (Doppler shift) of the emitted sound waves indicate both the velocity and the direction of the flowing blood. Also, the acoustic signal may be "gated" so that only those signals reflected at a particular distance from the emitter are detected. This allows one to compare the Doppler characteristics of blood flowing proximally or distally in the same artery. The TCD investigator can determine the linear blood flow velocity (LBFV) and direction of flowing blood in all the major intracerebral arteries based on their depth from the skin surface, the angle of insonation, and their anatomic relation to other arteries and arterial bifurcations.[29] The normal TCD waveform has a contour similar to the arterial blood pressure waveform. There is a rapid rise in velocity during systole, followed by a gradual decay of velocity during diastole. By analyzing and comparing the peak systolic LBFV (V_s), end diastolic LBFV (V_d), and mean LBFV (V_{mean}) of the TCD waveform, pulsatility and resistive indices (PI and RI) may be calculated. In the appropriate circumstances, PI and RI provide inferences about vascular elastance and resistance.

One important limitation of TCD is that its efficacy depends on the skills of the TCD investigator and interpreter. Because the technique is literally blind, a major source of error in repeated studies is the reproducibility of findings. Sorteberg et al[30] determined from normal subjects that a day-to-day LBFV variation must be greater than 20 percent to be considered significant at the 95 percent confidence level. An additional limitation is that the vessels are not imaged in two dimensions, as is commonly done with extracranial carotid duplex Doppler studies. Therefore, the actual vessel diameter is unknown. One common assumption, especially in TCD monitoring of vasospasm, is that any change in LBFV is due to a change in vessel diameter, but this is not always true. Changes in LBFV are actually due to changes in vascular resistance, which, in the cranium, may result either from changes of vessel diameter or from changes in ICP.[31]

In the ICU, TCD is a useful monitoring technique. It can be performed quickly at the bedside with minimal interference in patient care, and can be repeated as often as necessary. If desired, the TCD probe can be held in position by a head band for continuous monitoring. By properly obtaining the LBFV, RI, or PI of intracranial and extracranial arteries and performing arterial compression tests when appropriate, one may monitor the development of vasospasm,[32 to 34] the pattern of collateral circulation through the circle of Willis,[35] the state of cerebral arterial patency during thrombolytic therapy,[36,37] or the development of brain death.[38,39] TCD has been advocated as both a screening and a monitoring technique for elevated ICP,[34,40-42] but it is inaccurate when ICP is low and when patients have segmental arterial constriction, such as vasospasm or vascular stenosis. Klingelhöfer et al[34] studied the problem of patients with both vasospasm and elevated ICP and determined that ICP is less than 20 mmHg and that LBFV changes reflect changes in vessel diameter when the calculated Pourcelot RI is less than 0.5. However, when RI is greater than 0.6 and LBFV is less than 150 cm/s, the ICP is usually greater than 20 mmHg. Despite these findings, TCD remains an insensitive monitor of ICP and should not be used as the sole monitoring technique.

CEREBRAL METABOLISM AND ELECTROPHYSIOLOGY

One criticism of monitoring ICP, CPP, or TCD waveforms is that they provide no direct information about the physiologic functioning of the central nervous system. Monitoring and manipulating these parameters alone allows one to provide a theoretic "best physiologic milieu" for brain function and resuscitation, but unless a response can be monitored by the clinical examination, the physiologic response of the brain is unknown. One method of assessing the adequacy of CPP and CBF is to measure the change of cerebral consumption of metabolic substrates in response to therapy. A more direct approach is to perform electrophysiologic monitoring with electroencephalography (EEG) or evoked potentials (EPs), which may allow on-line, real-time data that can be used to diagnose, monitor and change interventions, or predict outcome.

Cerebral Substrate Metabolism

Measurement of cerebral metabolic substrate consumption requires sampling of systemic arterial and jugular venous blood. Jugular venous blood may be obtained from a single lumen vascular catheter that has been inserted in the internal jugular vein in a retrograde fashion. To accomplish this, the neck is prepared in the usual sterile manner and the vein is localized, first with a small-gauge needle and then a large needle, through which a guide wire is passed cranially until slight resistance is felt.[43] Conscious patients may note ear pain when the wire or catheter reach the jugular bulb. The catheter is then passed over the guide wire, which is removed. Skull films are taken to confirm that the catheter tip is in the jugular bulb. The right jugular vein should be catheterized, as the bulk of venous outflow from the cerebral hemispheres drains via the superior sagittal sinus to the right transverse sinus and jugular vein.[44]

Measuring the arteriovenous difference of oxygen ($AVDO_2$) or lactate (AVDL) can provide information regarding the presence of cerebral ischemia associated with elevated ICP. When serial measurements of $AVDO_2$ reveal elevation above the normal range (5.0 to 9.8 vol %) in response to hyperventilation to treat elevated ICP, this suggests that cerebral vasoconstriction is severe enough to cause ischemia.[45] Cruz et al[46] monitored jugular bulb oxyhemoglobin saturation by fiber optic catheter oximetry and found that low jugular vein oxygen saturation ($SjvO_2$) suggesting oligemia was reversed by administration of intravenous mannitol, but Sheinberg et al[47] found that $SjvO_2$ desaturation was not an early indicator of elevated ICP and usually occurred after tentorial herniation. Fiber optic $SjvO_2$ monitoring did identify hypoperfusion caused by hypocarbia and by desaturations resulting from systemic hypotension or hypoxia, but nearly half of all desaturations were artifactual from catheter malpositioning.[47] Robertson and co-workers[48] found that the lactate-oxygen index ($LOI = -AVDL/AVDO_2$) was consistent with ischemia and infarction if it was greater than 0.08. Patients with an LOI less than 0.08 did not have ischemia, and their CBF pattern could be classified according to the $AVDO_2$. An $AVDO_2$ less than 1.3 $\mu mol/ml$ was consistent with hyperemia, $AVDO_2$ between 1.3 to 3.0 was consistent with normal CBF, and $AVDO_2$ greater than 3.0 was consistent with compensated hypoperfusion.

EEG

Standard EEG recording uses 23 scalp electrodes in the International 10-20 system, and an 8- or 16-channel recorder with paper output. The EEG waveforms are analyzed with respect to location, frequency, amplitude, variability, response to stimuli, symmetry, and pattern. Although it is a sensitive technique, the volume of recorded data may be overwhelming and difficult to interpret except in the hands of practiced electroencephalographers. From a practical standpoint in the ICU, continuous standard EEG is best used in the setting of status epilepticus, when it is important to view moment-to-moment changes as anticonvulsants are given, to detect subclinical seizures, and to monitor the onset of a burst-suppression pattern when barbiturate general anesthesia is used to treat seizures.[5,49–51]

In many other diseases, instantaneous, highly resolved EEG data are not necessary for monitoring. Computer-processed EEG techniques have been developed that reduce the EEG signals to a manageable, more easily interpretable form. The compressed spectral array (CSA) is a technique in which EEG signals from sequential epochs of 4 to 32 seconds are analyzed by fast Fourier transformation to reveal the relative power of the EEG in each part of the frequency spectrum.[52] Individual power spectra are plotted on the ordinate, and subsequent epochs are offset on the abscissa to produce a three-dimensional plot, in which changes in peak height from spectrum to spectrum represent change over time. CSA may be useful for predicting outcome of coma. Bricolo et al[52] found that mortality was 93 percent for patients with a slow monotonous pattern on CSA, 46 percent with an alternating pattern, and 28 percent for those with sleep rhythms.

Evoked Potentials

EPs are neuronal electrical potentials that are recorded following sensory stimulation. In the ICU, evoked potentials are routinely recorded from the somatosensory pathways (SEP) and the brainstem auditory pathways (BAEP). These EPs use the technique of repetitive stimulation and recording, with signal averaging of all recorded potentials. Signal averaging eliminates background noise and random electrical potentials from other generator sites in the central nervous system or peripheral nervous system from the recorded EP. The averaged EP shows positive or negative electrical potentials, or waves, that occur at reproducible intervals, or latencies, following the stimulus. EPs are characterized in terms of absolute latency, interpeak latency, and amplitude.

BAEPs are recorded by placing headphones on the patient's ears to provide repetitive click stimuli. Recording electrodes are placed at the external acoustic meatus and the vertex of the head. The BAEP consists of waves I to V, which are thought to be generated by the VIIIth nerve action potential, the cochlear nucleus, the superior olivary complex, the lateral lemniscus, and the inferior colliculus.[53] Thus the BAEP can assess and localize lesions in the brainstem from the pons to the midbrain; however, injury to cranial nerve VIII (e.g., petrous fracture) may alter or obliterate the entire BAEP, in which case its use is unreliable. The BAEP is relatively resistant to the effects of benzodiazepines, barbiturates, or muscle relaxants, which are used often in the ICU.[54,55]

The localizing ability of BAEP may be useful for either monitoring or outcome prediction. For example, in patients with elevated ICP, prolongation of the wave V latency, (which originates in the inferior colliculus) suggests midbrain compression and impending uncal herniation, but normalization does not correlate with clinical improvement.[56] Barelli et al[57] found that head-injured patients who had all five waves present, with either normal or prolonged central conduction time, generally had a good outcome, whereas those who had absence of all waves, waves III, IV and V, or waves IV and V, all died. Lindsay et al[58] found that of 23 head-injured patients with wave V absent, 17 died, 2 were in a persistent vegetative state, and 4 were severely disabled. The SEP N20 wave was also absent in those who died or were vegetative, and Lindsay et al conclude that the absence of both BAEP and SEP predicts a poor outcome. However, Lindsay's group also found that brain stem auditory conduction time (BCT, wave I to V interpeak latency) and SEP central conduction time (see below) were no better at predicting outcome than clinical indicators, including the Glasgow coma scale (GCS), pupil response, and eye movements.[58] They recommend that BAEP and SEP evaluation is justified only for patients who are paralyzed or sedated and cannot be examined. Karnaze et al[59] used a neurophysiologic coma scale (NPCS), which includes BAEPs, long-latency auditory EPs, GCS, age, and brain stem reflexes, to predict outcome after head injury and found that the NPCS did not falsely predict a poor outcome for any patient, as opposed to the GCS, which falsely predicted a poor outcome in 10 of 21 patients. In patients with spontaneous intracerebral hemorrhage, those with normal BAEPs made a good recovery, whereas those with bilateral pathologic BAEPs either died or were severely disabled.[60]

SEPs are recorded by stimulating the median nerves at the wrists and recording from electrodes over the cervical spine and the scalp, over the contralateral sensory cortex. Stimulation of the tibial nerve and placement of additional recording electrodes may be performed as clinically indicated. Commonly evaluated waves are N13 or N14, recorded from the cervical electrode, and N20 recorded from the scalp electrode. N13/N14 represent near-field potentials in the dorsal horn interneurons,[61] and N20 represents near-field potentials in the primary somatosensory cortex.[62] Both spinal and cortical components of the SEP are preserved in the presence of therapeutic barbiturate coma, but the cortical wave amplitude may be diminished and the latency delayed, particularly at higher doses.[54,55]

The central conduction time (CCT) is the interpeak latency between N13/N14 and N20 and represents the time required for the afferent volley to traverse the brainstem, thalamus, and thalamocortical radiations.[63] The duration of the CCT has been used for both monitoring purposes and outcome prediction. In head injury, Hume and Cant[64] found that 75 percent of patients with normal CCT within 3.5 days of injury made a good recovery (Glasgow outcome score), while Judson et al[65] reported that 87 percent with normal and symmetric CCT had a good recovery or moderate disability. Judson et al also found that 73 percent of patients with asymmetric CCTs or with a prolonged CCT on either side had the same favorable outcome and concluded that the presence or absence of a cortical potential is more important for outcome prediction than any change in the CCT. Lindsay et al[58] found that CCT correlated well with clinical assessment of patients, but assisted in outcome prediction only in those who were paralyzed or sedated and could not be examined.

Asymmetry of the SEP may correlate with focal neurological injury. Hume and Cant[63] noted that persistent asymmetry of CCT and N20 amplitude or unilateral absence of N20 predicted hemiplegia in head-injured patients. CCT has been found to fluctuate with focal neurological deficits associated with the delayed vasospasm of subarachnoid hemorrhage,[66] but its clinical use is limited unless frequent or continuous monitoring is performed.[67] When frequent SEPs were recorded in a laboratory model of unilateral subarachnoid hemorrhage and chronic vasospasm, CCT prolongation was found to represent critical changes in CBF. Takeuchi and co-workers[68] measured CBF and CCT in both cerebral hemispheres of cynomolgus monkeys 7 days after instillation of blood in the basal subarachnoid space on the right. The MABP was manipulated from 40 to 180 mmHg to determine pressure autoregulation. In the hemisphere with vasospasm, there was no pressure autoregulation, and MABP of 130 percent to 150 percent of baseline was required to maintain CBF equal to the unaffected hemisphere. CCT was prolonged in the hemisphere with vasospasm when MABP was 40 mmHg or when CBF was less than 20 ml/100 g/min. As long as CBF exceeded 20 ml/100 g/min in either hemisphere, CCT was constant, but as CBF fell below 20, CCT increased linearly.

The bilateral absence of cortical potentials (N20) is consistently associated with brain death or persistent vegetative state,[58,64,65] however, Lindsay's group[58] reported one such patient who subsequently recovered N20 and survived with a good outcome. N20 reflects only cortical activity, and it may be absent when cerebral or brainstem activity is preserved. Chancellor et al[69] found that the absence of P17, a thalamic far-field potential recorded from the cervical electrode, more specifically predicted clinical brain death than the absence of N20 did. When brainstem activity was clinically present or when EEG activity of cerebral origin was seen, P17 was intact bilaterally, but when clinical brain death was confirmed, P17 was always absent bilaterally. N20 was absent in about two-thirds of those with residual cerebral or brainstem activity and would have prematurely confirmed brain death in these patients who all eventually died, although one survived for 75 days.

SUMMARY

Many techniques for monitoring ICP and cerebral or cerebrovascular function in the ICU exist. Continuous, on-line monitoring is possible for ICP and CSA EEG, whereas intermittent, frequent monitoring is usually undertaken for TCD, cerebral substrate metabolism determination, standard EEG, BAEP, and SEP. Although these techniques may be useful in guiding cerebral resuscitation, they require considerable time for set-up, data collection, and interpretation. The efficient and easily repeatable neurological examination must not be overlooked as an important monitoring technique in the ICU, despite some limitations in unconscious patients.[58,70] Refinement of existing techniques and improvement of on line data collection, display, and computer-assisted interpretation will improve our ability to monitor important cerebral functions.

MANAGING ELEVATED
INTRACRANIAL PRESSURE

Measures for controlling ICP can be divided into those used to reverse critical elevations and frank herniation and those used to maintain ICP below critical threshold levels. As a general rule, we attempt to keep ICP less than 20 mmHg and CPP greater than 70 mmHg at all times. Rapidly acting measures include hyperventilation, osmotic diuretics, ventricular drainage, and small doses of barbiturates. Maintenance therapy includes fluid restriction and diuretics, sedation and paralysis, seizure prophylaxis, fever prevention, and proper patient positioning. When intracranial hypertension is refractory to standard therapy, barbiturate coma may sometimes be appropriate.

Hyperventilation is one of the most rapid techniques; it can reduce ICP in a matter of minutes. The resulting hypocarbia ($PaCO_2$ 25 ± 2 torr) causes cerebral vasoconstriction in intact brain, which reduces CBF and blood volume, which reduces ICP. The alkalosis caused by hypocarbia is responsible for the vasoconstriction, but its effect diminishes as systemic acid–base buffering mechanisms compensate. Thus, hyperventilation for more than 6 hours diminishes in effectiveness and may even be harmful.[71] Despite this loss of effect, hyperventilation should not be stopped suddenly, as a rapid rise of $PaCO_2$ will increase ICP as easily as a rapid reduction lowers it. Hyperventilation should be removed gradually by increasing $PaCO_2$ from 25 to 35 torr over 24 to 48 hours as the ICP and CPP permit. Once the $PaCO_2$ is near 35 torr, hyperventilation may be used again to treat subsequent ICP elevations.

Osmotic diuresis with mannitol is the next most rapid treatment for intracranial hypertensive crises. Like hyperventilation, its physiologic effect is on intact brain. Mannitol creates an osmotic gradient across the blood–brain barrier. Water moves from brain to the intravascular compartment, reducing intracranial volume and, hence, ICP. In the acute situation, doses of 0.25 to 1.0 g/kg IV have roughly equivalent effects on ICP; however, the administration of larger doses may make the ICP less responsive to subsequent mannitol usage.[72] Mannitol's effect on ICP occurs in 10 to 20 minutes, and although rapid administration is desirable, mannitol can cause hemolysis if given too rapidly. Generally, injecting the dose over 10 minutes lowers ICP rapidly but has little risk of hemolysis. Infusion of mannitol solution will also transiently expand the intravascular volume. This may cause a brief increase of cerebral blood volume, which can cause the ICP to rise briefly before it falls. In rare instances, mannitol does not lower ICP or actually causes a persistent elevation. This is usually an indication of severe, diffuse cerebral injury and should prompt consideration of more aggressive therapy.

We prefer to reserve mannitol for acute intervention. Continuous infusion or regularly scheduled doses can be difficult to manage from the standpoint of fluid and electrolyte balance. Reduction of such therapy is often prolonged, because ICP can increase if the intravascular osmolarity is reduced too quickly.

Emergent ventricular drainage can be life-saving, as previously mentioned. Most neurosurgeons desire a computed tomography (CT) scan before inserting an IVC, because intracranial compartmental shifts can distort the ventricular position in relation to the external anatomic landmarks. Once a patient has been stabilized with hyperventilation and mannitol, a trip to the CT scanner may be indicated to determine whether an IVC can be inserted and whether a surgically correctable lesion exists.

Brief elevations of ICP often occur in the course of routine ICU care in patients with poor intracranial compliance. Endotracheal suction, changing the patient's position, and vascular catheter insertion are common procedures that elevate ICP. The risk of these brief elevations is that they may coalesce into sustained elevations that compromise cerebral perfusion. Prophylactic therapy can prevent this from happening. Prior to these common stimulating events, we often administer 50 to 100 mg thiopental or 75 to 100 mg lidocaine IV. Before endotracheal suction, additional hyperventilation may be used to attenuate the ICP response. Although these prophylactic measures are not always necessary, it is necessary to be aware of the risk of ICP elevation in response to routine care, and to be prepared to recognize and treat it.

Fluid restriction and diuretic therapy are the mainstays of ICP maintenance. Maintenance fluids are restricted to half the normal daily volume. Loop diuretics (furosemide) and carbonic anhydrase inhibitors (acetazolamide) can be used individually or combined to improve water clearance from the brain. They promote free water clearance by the kidney, increase serum osmolarity, and reduce CSF production. Acetazolamide can counteract the hyperchloremic metabolic alkalosis that furosemide can cause. The initial therapeutic goal with these agents is to elevate serum osmolarity to 300 to 310 mosm without reducing intravascular circulating volume (isovolemic hyperosmolarity). Therefore, free water losses must be replaced with isotonic solutions. The risk of volume depletion with diuretic therapy is that hypotension may ensue and compromise cerebral perfusion. Normal saline (0.9 percent NaCl), with KCl as indicated, is the most appropriate replacement crystalloid solution. Plasma or albumen solutions usually contain 140 ± 5 mEq NaCl and thus offer the potential advantage of providing both oncotic and osmotic particles to keep water in the intravascular space. Blood should be given to keep the hematocrit 30 ± 5 percent. Chronic diuretic therapy can deplete systemic electrolytes, such as potassium, magnesium, or phosphate, and these should be monitored daily and replaced when necessary.

Diuretic and dehydration therapy may last for 2 weeks while cerebral compliance returns to normal. Furosemide and acetazolamide are probably more effective at controlling ICP for long periods, because there is no tolerance to their diuretic effect, and they may decrease the risk of rebound cerebral edema from mannitol usage. An additional method of restricting fluids and providing adequate nutrition is to use high-calorie (2 kcal/ml) enteral feeding solutions.

Corticosteroids are not routinely given to reduce intracranial hypertension caused by head injury. If ICP is elevated as a result of tumor or abscess, large doses of dexamethasone (24 to 80 mg/day IV or enterally in adults) can help to maintain ICP below critical thresholds.

Agitation, coughing, resisting mechanical ventilation, and pain can elevate ICP. Narcotics (fentanyl or morphine) and nondepolarizing muscle relaxants (e.g., pancuronium) will not affect cerebrovascular resistance or reactivity and will not elevate ICP as long as $PaCO_2$ and PaO_2 are maintained with the ventilator. Although it has commonly been suggested that these agents obscure the clinical evaluation, their effects may be reversed in a matter of minutes if neurological assessment is needed, and their use is often more beneficial than detrimental.

Seizures cause a profound elevation of CBF, blood volume, and ICP in patients, whether they are paralyzed or not. Status epilepticus can cause further cerebral injury, or death by itself. We prefer to use phenytoin for seizure prevention, because it may be given either intravenously or enterally and does not sedate patients as phenobarbital can.

Fever can exacerbate ICP, and aggressive treatment with acetaminophen, aspirin, or a cooling blanket can be effective. Patients should not be chilled to the point of shivering, because this can elevate ICP. Positioning is another important aspect of ICP maintenance. The head should not be turned to the side because jugular venous drainage can be obstructed, causing ICP elevation. For most patients, elevating the head of the bed 20 to 30 degrees is beneficial, although in some instances head elevation can impair CPP.[73]

High-dose barbiturate therapy is an appropriate treatment for elevated ICP in those patients refractory to conventional management. Another indication is cerebral $AVDO_2$ evidence of cerebral ischemia in response to hyperventilation or dehydration. Ten to 15 percent of head-injured patients are in this category, and approximately half will respond to barbiturate coma. High-dose barbiturate therapy is the administration of a general anesthetic in the ICU. It is complicated and requires a skilled intensive care team capable of managing an anesthetized, critically ill patient for prolonged periods.

We prefer to use pentobarbital because it has no active metabolites and has a predictable half-life of about 24 hours, and because serum levels may be determined. Therapeutic levels are 25 to 40 mg/L. Cardiovascular collapse should be anticipated at the onset of therapy, particularly because virtually all patients are maximally dehydrated when barbiturate coma is begun. Vasoconstrictors, inotropes, and volume expansion may be needed rapidly, and all patients should have a pulmonary artery balloon catheter in place to guide hemodynamic management as barbiturate therapy is begun. With these precautions, a pentobarbital loading dose of 36 mg/kg may be given without risking CPP. Therapeutic coma abolishes the neurological examination, and electrophysiologic monitoring is mandatory. EEG will show a burst suppression pattern when the pentobarbital level is 30 to 40 mg/L. This is associated with a maximal reduction of both cerebral metabolic rate of oxygen consumption ($CMRO_2$) and ICP. If ICP cannot be reduced with barbiturates when a burst suppression pattern is present, higher doses are unlikely to be effective, and withdrawal of therapy should be considered.

CEREBRAL RESUSCITATION

BRAIN INJURY

Brain injury always has been defined by the type of pathologic insult. A major assumption has been that injury processes are different and relate to the underlying initial insult. Several broad categories of injury include global ischemia, focal ischemia, trauma, acute masses, and metabolic injuries. Global ischemia is defined as a complete cessation of blood flow to the entire brain. Clinically, this most often occurs with cardiac arrest, and therefore is associated with multiorgan circulatory failure. Focal ischemia is characterized as complete circulatory impairment of a small region of cerebral tissue, usually a region supplied by a first- or second-order branch of the circle of Willis. It is important to recognize that global and focal ischemia may be incomplete (i.e., the injury can be a decrease of blood flow below the threshold necessary to maintain cellular function, but not complete circulatory standstill).

The third category of injury is trauma. The simplest definition of trauma is brain contusion, which usually consists of a mechanical component that distends brain tissue both at the surface and deeper at several key structures. Contusion injury is also associated with mechanical forces that disrupt single axons and tracts of white matter. There is a delayed component of contusion injury that consists of reperfusion and ischemic insults.

The fourth type of injury is the acute mass. Here the injury is characterized by direct trauma to brain tissue. The amount of trauma is related to the rate of growth of the acute mass and to the amount of displacement of brain structures. Examples include spontaneous intracerebral hemorrhage and epidural hematoma.

Metabolic injury is the fifth type and is a more diverse category. It includes the excess accumulation of substances toxic to neuronal cellular activity and the insufficient supply of specific chemical entities necessary for normal neuronal cellular activity. Renal and hepatic encephalopathies, hypoxia, and exogenous neuronal toxins, such as cyanide, are examples. Recently, the notion of endogenous intoxication has greatly influenced our thinking about brain injury. In distinction to many exogenous metabolic factors, endogenous toxins such as glutamate and glycine have now been implicated in the production of delayed, possibly reversible, damage to selective neuronal populations.

Two additional types of injury are those caused by reperfusion and inflammation. Both are reactive injury processes, requiring primary events such as ischemia or infection to trigger a pathophysiologic response that is poorly contained, and hence toxic, to adjacent normal tissues.

The precise mechanism by which each of these injury categories promotes cellular damage and loss of neurological function remains incompletely explored, although partial characterizations of injurious factors have been made with animal models for each of these categories. Similarly, the precise mechanisms of injury for the reactive processes, reperfusion, and inflammation remain incompletely characterized. Thus, a medical knowledge base needed for specific pharmacologic manipulation of these injuries is not presently available. Similarly, a detailed anatomic characterization of injury processes and the evolution of cell death is only partially understood. Therefore, the rationale for selection of specific surgical treatments also remains incompletely justified. It is from this perspective that we discuss brain monitoring and resuscitation.

CARDIAC ARREST: THE MODEL FOR IDEAL CEREBRAL RESUSCITATION

Reversal

Cerebral resuscitation has been narrowly described as the reversal of clinical death in the situation of cardiac arrest. The comatose patient who has suffered a complete cardiopulmonary arrest probably comprises the single largest subset of patients in this category. These are ideal patients for the reversal of clinical death with pharmacologic and other therapeutic strategies. Unfortunately, the incidence of hypoxic-ischemic neurological damage, and the eventual mortality, remains unchanged over the last three decades.[74] Furthermore, barbiturates and calcium antagonists have each been tested as cerebral resuscitation agents in clinical trials and shown not to have efficacy.[75,76]

Serious hypoxic-ischemic insults can be defined as those representing greater than 10 minutes of complete global ischemia. When the duration of cardiac arrest is unknown, an alternative criterion of prolonged coma (>6 hours after resuscitation) can be used to select patients who are at high risk for severe neurological sequelae. Evaluations of groups of cardiac arrest patients have suggested that 80 percent to 90 percent of those with serious hypoxic-ischemic insults will die, and a small minority will survive with severe neurological injury.[74–76] The initial neurological examination and repeat evaluations are helpful in assessing whether an individual patient is recovering or demonstrating signs of severe injury. The absence of brain stem function at 6 and 24 hours after arrest represents a constellation of findings highly predictive of death or severe injury. Levy and co-workers[74] defined specific predictive values to discrete parts of the neurological examination based on their evaluation of a cohort of comatose patents. At 24 hours, predictors of a poor prognosis are a motor response no better than flexor and the absence of spontaneous or roving eye movements. Signs predicting a good prognosis at 24 hours are a motor response of simple withdrawal or better and the presence of eye opening. We find these signs helpful in developing a prognosis for patient's families. It should be qualified that the validity of these findings has not been prospectively tested.

Prophylaxis/Prevention

A major constraint in the resuscitation of these patients is the inability to treat them prior to the time of injury. Animal models suggest a greater potential benefit when pretreatment is given. Although pharmacologic prophylaxis is often unattainable for cardiac arrest, the recent development of automatic implantable defibrillator devices has the potential to prevent many patients from succumbing to global hypoxic-ischemic cerebral injury.[77]

PRACTICAL RESUSCITATION PARADIGMS IN OTHER FORMS OF CEREBRAL INJURY

Because of the failure of these treatments to alter the outcome after cardiac arrest, a wider definition of resuscitation is needed if monitoring activities are to predicate clinically effective treatments. A broader definition of cerebral resuscitation must therefore include all those clinical types of brain injury for which intervention has clear benefit. This group of injuries includes closed head injury, acute intracranial masses, subarachnoid hemorrhage, status epilepticus, and a limited number of cerebrovascular syndromes, with sagittal sinus and basilar artery thrombosis being the two most discrete. Each of these is a clear, diagnostically defined disease for which natural history and outcome information is known.[78,79] As pathophysiologic processes, they share a common theme of primary injury and delayed secondary injury. Controlled studies of each of these diseases have shown the effects of intervention on either intermediate physiologic variables or outcome variables that are clinical markers of desirable long-term outcomes.

Thus, the study of brain injury has necessarily led to therapies that focus on preventing further damage or limiting the progression of damage.[1,80–86] The cerebral monitoring techniques described in the first part of this chapter are directed at the goal of preventing further injury from any of these harmful processes. A secondary goal is to assess the efficacy and toxicity of individual therapies, allowing them to be adjusted in accordance with the evolution of the patient's disease process. In the remainder of this chapter, we review cerebral resuscitation options for common cerebral diseases by identifying both resuscitation and prophylactic therapies when they exist. The specific therapeutic strategies fall into three general categories: preventing cerebral hypoperfusion, minimizing excitation injury, and re-establishing perfusion to already ischemic tissue. In its most generic sense, this is the science of cerebral resuscitation.

Cerebral Ischemia After Cardio/cerebrovascular Surgery

Reversal Neurological assessment after cardiac surgery often is delayed, which prohibits identification of ischemia during a time frame that allows for reversal. Thrombectomy, anticoagulation, and immediate operation for internal carotid occlusion have been associated with reversal of neurological deficits in some, but by no means all, patients.

Prophylaxis/prevention Prophylactic blood pressure and shunting measures for occlusive vascular disease have not been shown to have significant efficacy. An exception to this statement may be the empiric use of hypothermia in situations of circulatory arrest. Here, historic evidence suggests the ability of hypothermia less than 26°C to decrease the incidence of postoperative ischemic deficits. Animal models have suggested potential benefits of small reductions in brain temperature from 38° to 33°C.[87] Human data testing the benefit of such treatments are not available currently.

Stroke/Transient Ischemic Attack

Reversal Reversal of focal cerebral ischemia is rarely achieved in middle cerebral artery territory occlusions.[88] Recent trials of thrombolysis, although promising, do not demonstrate a clearly efficacious regimen. However, two other disease situations, basilar artery occlusion and sagittal sinus occlusion, have been associated with reversible ischemic deficits. For basilar territorial ischemia with demonstrated basilar artery occlusion, thrombolysis performed within the first 12 hours of symptoms appears to be associated with improved morbidity and mortality if recanalization can be shown. Recanalization in a large cohort of patients could only be accomplished in 50 percent of the cases.[85] Thus, this still remains a disease with high morbidity and mortality. The frequent morbidity associated with basilar artery occlusion and the improvement of treated patients over historical controls suggests significant potential for reversibility if the appropriate selection criteria can be defined. As in all other forms of cerebral resuscitation, the role of reperfusion injury in this disease has not been investigated.

Cerebral venous occlusion provides a less acute model of injury. Patients with this disorder frequently present with up to 30 days of symptoms. They probably experience a gradual decline in CPP, and a subgroup may experience multiple small parenchymal hemorrhages. Where the venous obstructive lesion extends to the deep venous system draining the brainstem, altered level of consciousness and cranial nerve findings are part of a more rapid deterioration. Both heparin and urokinase have been shown to produce recanalization of the sagittal sinus. A recent controlled study showed improved neurological performance and mortality for a heparin-treated group of patients when compared with placebo.[7] When ICP elevation is severe, there may be a role for more aggressive management of cranial vault problems such as impaired CPP.[89]

Prophylaxis/prevention Cerebral ischemia from occlusive vascular disease is remediable if long-term prophylaxis is undertaken for the disease categories of nonvalvular atrial fibrillation, high-grade carotid stenosis, and transient ischemic attack.

The issue of optimal control of blood pressure in the hypertensive acutely ill neurological patient, and particularly in patients with acute stroke, is often discussed. Long-term antihypertensive prophylaxis is best deferred until the acute phase of the illness has remitted. There is no objective evidence that such therapy benefits these patients, and there are many reports of cerebral ischemia provoked by aggressive antihypertensive use. We do not recommend the use of antihypertensive agents as initial treatment for severe blood pressure elevation. Rather, we advocate the use of appropriate analgesics and sedatives to minimize pain and agitation, which are usually the causes of hypertension in the ICU. If elevation of MABP greater than 135 mmHg occurs, if cardiac function is impaired, or if extreme blood pressure lability exists, labetalol or nitroprusside can be used cautiously in gradually increasing doses. Reducing MABP to 115 to 125 mmHg is reasonable in the setting of possible cerebral ischemia. We discontinue these agents if neurological signs worsen, as they can produce elevated ICP or progressive ischemia. This is especially important when using nitroprusside or other nitrate agents, such as nitroglycerin, in the setting of elevated ICP. These agents are best used when ICP and CPP are monitored. Nitroprusside and nitroglycerin dilate cerebral vessels and can cause an increase of cerebral blood volume and elevation of ICP. Thus, nitroprusside and nitroglycerin can doubly compromise CPP by lowering MABP and raising ICP.

Subarachnoid Hemorrhage/Vasospasm

Reversal For the gradually progressive global and focal deficits of vasospasm, hypervolemic hypertensive therapy appears to produce clear reversal of apparently fixed neurological signs. The strongest evidence for benefit of blood pressure and blood volume manipulations rests with inadvertent single patient cross-over design observations in which volume and pressure components of treatment have been discontinued and neurological findings return. Carefully collated hypervolemic hypertensive therapy data suggest improvement in neurological status can be linked to this manipulation.[6] For individuals who tolerate hemodynamic manipulations poorly, angioplasty has been recommended.[90,91] Here, case series suggest a 70 percent improvement rate associated with dilation of involved vessels. Data from a controlled trial of this treatment are not available presently.

In treating symptomatic vasospasm, we advocate the use of isotonic fluids, either normal saline or plasma or albumin solutions, as volume expanders to increase the pulmonary capillary wedge pressure to 15 ± 3 mmHg. We also use dopamine and phenylephrine to increase MABP to 125 ± 5 mmHg. This can usually be accomplished with 10 to 15 μg/kg/min of dopamine or 10 to 40 μg/kg/min of phenylephrine. We attempt to raise perfusion pressure at the earliest sign of neurological impairment, which is usually an alteration of level of consciousness or of motor performance.

Prophylaxis/prevention Subarachnoid hemorrhage presents the disease process best suited for prophylaxis and resuscitation. In large part, this is due to prior efforts to define the natural history of the disease and its treatments. Furthermore, there are many successfully demonstrated treatments for subarachnoid hemorrhage. Finally, a therapeutic advantage exists with vasospasm-induced cerebral injury because it occurs gradually compared with the ischemic deficits of stroke or closed head injury.[92]

After a patient experiences acute subarachnoid hemorrhage, further brain injury is caused either by recurrent bleeding or delayed ischemia of vasospasm. Early surgical correction of the vessel wall defect is the best way to minimize the risk of further brain damage from arterial bleeding. This role for early surgery has been advocated at many medical centers. Although older studies in the subacute time frames of 0 to 3, 3 to 7, and more than 7 days do not show a benefit for early surgery,[93] most centers that operate in the first 24 hours after hemorrhage have shown improvement compared with historical morbidity.[94]

With adequate vascular reconstruction, the only remaining major cause of cerebral injury is the vasospasm syndrome. The role of volume depletion in initiating this syndrome has been defined by Widjicks et al.[95] More recently, Soloman et al[94] showed the benefit of early volume loading as part of presurgical and postsurgical management. This maneuver decreases the incidence of vasospasm. Although the precise mechanism by which this works is not clear, Diringer et al[96] showed that moderate volume loading blocks the anticipated decline in plasma volume, and Awad et al[6] showed that blood pressure elevation can minimize cerebral ischemic symptoms.

A different class of agents, the calcium antagonists, has been shown to have cerebral protective effects when administered prior to the occurrence of ischemic injury. In this setting, the expected 20 percent incidence of permanent ischemic deficits is reduced to approximately 10 percent. These findings were initially described by Allen et al[97] and have subsequently been repeated in four other double-blind placebo-controlled studies, including a large cohort studied by Pickard et al.[98]

Head Injury

Reversal   Acute mass effects are seen with subdural and epidural hematomas, cerebellar hematoma, and occasionally with other masses causing acute obstructive hydrocephalus. These patients present with a rapidly progressive loss of consciousness and clear evidence of brainstem compression, usually with ventricular dilation with or without cranial nerve palsy. In this setting, impaired airway reflexes and obtundation are often associated with aspiration and hypoxia. Rapid sequence intubation with succinylcholine and low-dose thiopental prevents aspiration and permits rapid hyperventilation. Emergent ventricular drainage can lead to a marked decline in ICP and sometimes a sudden, remarkable return to consciousness. Where a posterior fossa mass has led to aqueductal obstruction, ventricular drainage can be closely coupled with surgical correction of the mass effect. By minimizing the period of impaired CPP and removing direct brainstem compression, both coma and neurological deficits may be reversed. Case series suggest that early aggressive treatment for these mass lesions will produce a 50 percent survival rate. This appears to be a significant improvement from historical controls. Several clinical factors appear to indicate a lower likelihood of successful resuscitation. These include existence of a posterior fossa mass larger than 3 cm in diameter; complete absence of brainstem reflexes including BAEP; and prolonged periods of brainstem compression before therapeutic intervention.

Prophylaxis/prevention Closed head injury represents the most common form of brain injury. Prophylactic efforts for cerebral contusion most likely provide significant benefit to the injury victim. This injury is complex, with components of direct trauma and reperfusion injury. Delayed edema occurs progressively for several days after the initial injury. Elevated ICP, as a consequence of edema, may lead to transient or permanent impairment of cerebral perfusion. Prophylactic monitoring and treatments aimed at decreasing brain water content are probably efficacious therapeutic measures. Although they have not been directly linked to improved outcomes as single modalities, ICP monitoring and dehydration therapy with free water limitation, diuretics, and osmotic agents are a part of the general medical regimen in most head injury centers reporting improved mortality and morbidity. The use of these agents individually and in combination is clearly associated with decreased ICP in individual patients.

Conversely, a distinct subpopulation of patients do not demonstrate decreases of ICP below 30 mmHg when treated with maximal passive and active dehydration regimens. When these elevations are protracted, severe compromise of intracranial perfusion is possible either from intermittent hypotension, with impairment of the CPP, or from transient elevation of ICP, as occurs with the Lundberg A and B waves. This situation is relatively uncommon (10 percent of all brain injuries) and represents the most severely injured subgroup of traumatic brain injury. The failure to respond to prophylactic measures can be shown clearly with ICP monitoring. Jugular bulb oxygenation monitoring may improve our ability to diagnose patients with CPP-induced cerebral perfusion impairment.[45-48, 99] When ICP is poorly controlled, an effort to define unrecognized mass lesions remediable by surgery should be undertaken. Either CT scanning or magnetic resonance imaging provides an adequate screen for intercurrent cerebral hematoma. Without evidence of such a lesion, high-dose barbiturate therapy will provide an opportunity for increased ICP control. The value of this treatment in improving morbidity and mortality has been shown recently by Eisenberg et al.[10]

The intermittent presence of A and B waves suggests that sequential ischemia and reperfusion may occur multiple times during the course of a closed head injury. Although animal models have shown the importance of reperfusion injury mechanisms, the role for pharmacologic protection from reperfusion injury has yet to be demonstrated in this illness. Currently, a trial of superoxide dismutase, an enzyme that decreases the generation of free radicals during reperfusion, is underway. Similarly, the role of brain temperature and excitotoxins has only begun to be explored in animal models of this disease. A final pharmacologic agent of some significance in animal models is the opiate antagonists. Here, the κ subpopulation of opiate receptors appears to undergo significant stimulation after head injury.[100] Some improvement in animal performance and histologic damage scores is seen with pre- and postinjury treatment with the κ antagonist drugs, but human data for head injury are not available. The opiate antagonists have not been shown to be effective in spinal cord injury or in small groups of cerebral ischemic injury patients.

Status Epilepticus

Reversal Status epilepticus represents another brain injury with a clearly reversible component. The progression from single seizures to prolonged ictal discharges and brain injury is well documented in animal models. The apparent combination of increased excitation from elevated extracellular glutamate concentrations and decreased inhibition from decreased γ-aminobutyric acid (GABA) concentrations may have a direct effect on the extent of cell death in both status epilepticus and cerebral ischemia. Extrapolations of animal work to humans suggest a 30-minute window for limiting neuronal damage.[101] A controlled study is now underway to define the optimum regimen for electrophysiologic suppression of ictal discharges.[102] The linking of treatment to outcome has been more difficult in status epilepticus, as both the etiology of the seizures and the presence of concurrent medical complications have limited our ability to perform controlled studies. For patients refractory to the combination of benzodiazepines and phenytoin, high-dose barbiturate therapy has been recommended with significant success.[3–5] Neither the mechanism of action nor the ability to reverse or limit the progression of injury has been defined for these agents. Animal models strongly suggest that augmentation of GABA-ergic activity and blockade of glutamatergic activity are of significant theoretic value. A recent case series suggests some value to the augmentation of GABA activity.[103]

Metabolic

Reversal Reversal of hypoglycemic coma and/or focal deficits occurs on replacement of glucose deficits. Duration of hypoglycemic reversibility is poorly understood and is most likely a complex product of metabolic rate and metabolic compensation with alternate fuel sources. Reversal of hepatic encephalopathy with benzodiazepine antagonists has now been accomplished in small groups of patients. Again, injury thresholds have not been investigated. The benefits of this treatment in terms of patient outcome remain to be demonstrated.

Prophylaxis/prevention Dehydration appears to be well tolerated by the central nervous system without long-term consequences. However, rapid swings in hydration status are associated with significant demyelination. Historical data strongly suggest that rapid shifts from normal osmolar status to severe hypo-osmolality and shifts from hypo-osmolality to hyperosmolality may be associated with irreversible glial cell damage. The best available data indicate that increases of more than 40 mosm in 24 hours is accompanied with a significant incidence of demyelination.[104–106] For the hyperosmolar patient who is not seizing, slow correction of hyponatremia at the rate of less than 0.5 mEq/h or less than 1 mosm/h is recommended.

SUMMARY

Cerebral resuscitation in contemporary practice comprises techniques for preventing secondary neurological injury. The reversal of primary neurological injury remains in the realm of the researcher. As the pathophysiological mechanisms of primary injury and cell death are better understood, specific pharmacologic and surgical therapies may be developed that can produce true cerebral resuscitation.

REFERENCES

1. Saul TG, Ducker TB: Effect of intracranial pressure monitoring and aggressive treatment on mortality in severe head injury. J Neurosurg 56:498, 1982
2. Sarnaik AP, Kopec J, Moylan P et al: Role of aggressive intracranial pressure control in management of pediatric craniocerebral gunshot wounds with unfavorable features. J Trauma 29:1434, 1989
3. Rashkin MD, Youngs C, Penovich P: Pentobarbital treatment of refractory status epilepticus. Neurology 37:500, 1987
4. Lowenstein DH, Aminoff MJ, Simon RP: Barbiturate anesthesia in the treatment of status epilepticus: clinical experience with 14 patients. Neurology 38:395, 1988
5. VanNess PC: Pentobarbital and EEG burst suppression in treatment of status epilepticus refractory to benzodiazepines and phenytoin. Epilepsia 31:61, 1990
6. Awad IA, Carter LP, Spetzler RF et al: Clinical vasospasm after subarachnoid hemorrhage: response to hypervolemic hemodilution and arterial hypertension. Stroke 18:365, 1987
7. Kassel NF, Peerless SJ, Durward QJ et al: Treatment of ischemic deficits from vasospasm with intravascular volume expansion and induced arterial hypertension. Neurosurgery 11:337, 1982
8. Guillaume J, Janny P: Manométrie intracranienne continue. Intérêt de la méthode et premiers résultats. Rev Neurol (Paris) 84:131, 1954
9. Lundberg N: Continuous recording and control of ventricular fluid pressure in neurosurgical practice. Acta Psychiatr Neurol Scand Suppl 149:1, 1960
10. Eisenberg HM, Frankowski RF, Contant CF et al: High-dose barbiturate control of elevated intracranial pressure in patients with severe head injury. J Neurosurg 69:15, 1988
11. Marshall LF, Shapiro HM, Rauscher et al: Pentobarbital therapy for intracranial hypertension in metabolic coma. Reye's syndrome. Crit Care Med 6:1, 1978
12. McPherson RW, Koehler RC, Traystman RJ: Effect of jugular venous pressure on cerebral autoregulation in dogs. Am J Physiol 255 (Heart Circ Physiol 24):H1516, 1988
13. Tasker RC, Matthew DJ, Helms P et al: Monitoring in non-traumatic coma. Part I: invasive intracranial measurements. Arch Dis Child 63:888, 1988
14. McGillicuddy JE: Cerebral protection: pathophysiology and treatment of increased intracranial pressure. Chest 87:85, 1985
15. Helfaer MA, Kirsch JR: Intracranial vault pathophysiology. Crit Care Rep 1:12, 1989
16. Öhrström JK, Skou JK, Ejlertsen T et al: Infected ventriculostomy: bacteriology and treatment. Acta Neurochir (Wien) 100:67, 1989

17. Mayhall CG, Archer NH, Lamb A et al: Ventriculostomy-related infections. N Engl J Med 310:553, 1984
18. Smith RW, Alksne JF: Infections complicating the use of external ventriculostomy. J Neurosurg 44:567, 1976
19. Mendelow AD, Rowan JO, Murray L et al: A clinical comparison of subdural screw pressure measurements with ventricular pressure. J Neurosurg 58:45, 1983
20. Weaver DD, Winn HR, Jane JA: Differential intracranial pressure in patients with unilateral mass lesions. J Neurosurg 565:660, 1982
21. Yano M, Ikeda Y, Kobayashi S et al: Intracranial pressure in head-injured patients with various intracranial lesions is identical throughout the supratentorial intracranial compartment. Neurosurgery 21:688, 1987
22. Johnston IH, Rowan JO: Raised intracranial pressure and cerebral blood flow. J Neurol Neurosurg Psychiatry 37:585, 1974
23. Barnett GH, Chapman PH: Insertion and care of intracranial pressure monitoring devices. p. 43. In Ropper AH, Kennedy SK (eds): Neurological and Neurosurgical Intensive Care. 2nd Ed. Aspen Publishers, Rockville, MD, 1988
24. Crutchfield JS, Narayan RK, Robertson CS et al: Elevation of a fiberoptic intracranial pressure monitor. J Neurosurg 72:482, 1990
25. Chambers IR, Mendelow AD, Sinar EJ et al: A clinical evaluation of the Camino subdural screw and ventricular monitoring kits. Neurosurgery 26:421, 1990
26. Ostrup RC, Luerssen TG, Marshall LF et al: Continuous monitoring of intracranial pressure with a miniaturized fiberoptic device. J Neurosurg 67:206, 1987
27. Schickner DJ, Young RF: Intracranial pressure monitoring: fiberoptic monitor compared with the ventricular catheter. Surg Neurol 27:251, 1992
28. Aaslid R, Markwalder T, Nornes H: Noninvasive transcranial Doppler ultrasound recording of flow velocities in basal cerebral arteries. J Neurosurg 57:769, 1982
29. Ringelstein EB, Kahlscheuer B, Niggemeyer E et al: Transcranial Doppler sonography: anatomical landmarks and normal velocity values. Ultrasound Med Biol 16:745, 1990
30. Sorteberg W, Langmoen IA, Lindegaard K-F et al : Side-to-side differences and day-to-day variations of transcranial Doppler parameters in normal subjects. J Ultrasound Med 9:403, 1990
31. Aaslid R, Lindegaard K-F: Cerebral hemodynamics. p. 80. In Aaslid R (ed): Transcranial Doppler Sonography. Springer-Verlag, New York, 1986
32. Lindegaard K-F, Nornes H, Bakke SJ et al: Cerebral vasospasm diagnosis by means of angiography and blood velocity measurements. Acta Neurochir (Wien) 100:12, 1989
33. Sekhar LN, Wechsler LR, Yonas H et al: Value of transcranial Doppler examination in the diagnosis of cerebral vasospasm after subarachnoid hemorrhage. Neurosurgery 22:813, 1988
34. Klingelhöfer J, Sander D, Holzgraefe M et al: Cerebral vasospasm evaluated by transcranial Doppler ultrasonography at different intracranial pressures. J Neurosurg 75:752, 1991
35. Lindegaard K-F, Bakke SJ, Grolimund P et al: Assessment of intracranial hemodynamics in carotid artery disease by transcranial Doppler ultrasound. J Neurosurg 63:890, 1985
36. Karnik R, Stelzer P, Slany J: Transcranial Doppler sonography monitoring of local intra-arterial thrombolysis in acute occlusion of the middle cerebral artery. Stroke 23:284, 1992

37. Razumovsky A YE, Hanley DF, Willliams MA et al: TCD in acute brain stem stroke. Stroke 23:470, 1992 (abstract)

38. Hassler W, Steinmetz H, Gawlowski J: Transcranial Doppler ultrasonography in raised intracranial pressure and in intracranial circulatory arrest. J Neurosurg 68:745, 1988

39. Hassler W, Steinmetz H, Pirschel J: Transcranial Doppler study of intracranial circulatory arrest. J Neurosurg 71:195, 1989

40. Chadduck WM, Crabtree HM, Blankenship JB et al: Transcranial Doppler ultrasonography for the evaluation of shunt malfunction in pediatric patients. Childs Nerv Syst 7:27, 1991

41. Klingelhöfer J, Conrad B, Benecke R et al: Evaluation of intracranial pressure from transcranial Doppler studies in cerebral disease. J Neurol 235:159, 1988

42. Aaslid R, Lundar T, Lindegaard K-F et al: Estimation of cerebral perfusion pressure from arterial blood pressure and transcranial Doppler recordings. p. 226. In Miller JD, Teasdale GM, Rowan JO (eds): Intracranial Pressure VI. Springer-Verlag Berlin, Heidelberg, 1986

43. Jakobsen M, Enevoldsen E: Retrograde catheterization of the right internal jugular vein for serial measurements of cerebral venous oxygen content. J Cereb Blood Flow Metab 9:717, 1989

44. Capra NF, Anderson KV: Anatomy of the cerebral venous system. p. 1. In Kapp JP, Schmidek HH (eds): The Cerebral Venous System and Its Disorders. Grune & Stratton, Orlando, FL, 1984

45. Obrist WD, Langfitt TW, Jaggi JL et al: Cerebral blood flow and metabolism in comatose patients with acute head injury. J Neurosurg 61:241, 1984

46. Cruz J, Miner ME, Allen SJ et al: Continuous monitoring of cerebral oxygenation in acute brain injury: assessment of cerebral hemodynamic reserve. Neurosurgery 29:743, 1991

47. Sheinberg M, Kanter MJ, Robertson CS et al: Continuous monitoring of jugular venous oxygen saturation in head-injured patients. J Neurosurg 76:212, 1992

48. Robertson CS, Narayan RK, Gokaslan ZL et al: Cerebral arteriovenous oxygen difference as an estimate of cerebral blood flow in comatose patients. J Neurosurg 70:222, 1989

49. Rashkin MD, Youngs C, Penovich P: Pentobarbital treatment of refractory status epilepticus. Neurology 37:500, 1987

50. Lowenstein DH, Aminoff MJ, Simon RP: Barbiturate anesthesia in the treatment of status epilepticus: clinical experience with 14 patients. Neurology 38:395, 1988

51. Tasker RC, Boyd SG, Harden A et al: EEG monitoring of prolonged thiopentone administration for intractable seizures and status epilepticus in infants and young children. Neuropediatrics 20:147, 1988

52. Bricolo A, Faccioli F, Grosslercher JC et al: Electrophysiological monitoring in the intensive care unit. Electroencephalogr Clin Neurophysiol 39(suppl.):255, 1987

53. Chiappa KH: Electrophysiologic monitoring. p. 129. In Ropper AH, Kennedy SK (eds): Neurological and Neurosurgical Intensive Care. 2nd Ed. Aspen Publishers, Rockville, MD, 1988

54. Drummond JC, Todd MM, Schubert A et al: Effect of the acute administration of high dose pentobarbital on human brain stem auditory and median nerve somatosensory evoked responses. Neurosurgery 20:830, 1987

55. Sutton LN, Frewen T, Marsh R et al: The effects of deep barbiturate coma on multimodality evoked potentials. J Neurosurg 57:178, 1982

56. Nagao S, Kuyama H, Honma Y et al: Prediction and evaluation of brainstem function by auditory brainstem responses in patients with uncal herniation. Surg Neurol 27:81, 1987
57. Barelli A, Valente MR, Clemente A et al: Serial multimodality-evoked potentials in severely head-injured patients: Diagnostic and prognostic implications. Crit Care Med 19:1374, 1991
58. Lindsay K, Pasaoglu A, Hirst D et al: Somatosensory and auditory brain stem conduction after head injury: a comparison with clinical features in prediction of outcome. Neurosurgery 26:278, 1990
59. Karnaze DS, Weiner JM, Marshall LF: Auditory evoked potentials in coma after closed head injury: a clinical-neurophysiologic coma scale for predicting outcome. Neurology 35:1122, 1985
60. Lumenta CB: Measurements of brain-stem auditory evoked potentials in patients with spontaneous intracerebral hemorrhage. J Neurosurg 60:548, 1984
61. Desmedt JE: Noninvasive analysis of the spinal cord generators activated by somatosensory input in man: near-field and farfield components. p. 45. In Creutzfeldt O, Schmidt RF, Willis WD (eds): Sensory-Motor Integration in the Nervous System. (Exp Brain Res Suppl 9.) Springer-Verlag Berlin, Heidelberg, 1984
62. Celesia GG: Somatosensory evoked potentials recorded directly from the human thalamus and Sm1 cortical area. Arch Neurol 36:399, 1979
63. Hume AL, Cant BR: Conduction time in central somatosensory pathways in man. Electroencephalogr Clin Neurophysiol 45:361, 1978
64. Hume AL, Cant BR: Central somatosensory conduction after head injury. Ann Neurol 10:411, 1981
65. Judson JA, Cant BR, Shaw NA: Early prediction of outcome from cerebral trauma by somatosensory evoked potentials. Crit Care Med 18:363, 1990
66. Symon L, Hargadine J, Zawirski M et al: Central conduction time as an index of ischaemia in subarachnoid haemorrhage. J Neurol Sci 44:95, 1979
67. Wang AD, Cone J, Symon L et al: Somatosensory evoked potential monitoring during the management of aneurysmal SAH. J Neurosurg 60:264, 1984
68. Takeuchi H, Handa Y, Kobayashi H et al: Impairment of cerebral autoregulation during the development of chronic cerebral vasospasm after subarachnoid hemorrhage in primates. Neurosurgery 28:41, 1991
69. Chancellor AM, Frith RW, Shaw NA: Somatosensory evoked potentials following severe head injury: loss of the thalamic potential with brain death. J Neurol Sci 87:255, 1988
70. Williams MA: Neurologic examination of critically ill patients. Crit Care Rep 1:52, 1989
71. Muizelaar JP, Marmarou A, Ward JD et al: Adverse effects of prolonged hyperventilation in patients with severe head injury: a randomized clinical trial. J Neurosurg 75:731, 1991
72. McGraw CP, Howard G: Effect of mannitol on increased intracranial pressure. Neurosurgery 13:269, 1983
73. Feldman Z, Kanter MJ, Robertson CS et al: Effect of head elevation on intracranial pressure, cerebral perfusion pressure, and cerebral blood flow in head-injured patients. J Neurosurg 76:207, 1992
74. Levy DE, Coronna JJ, Singer BH et al: Predicting outcome from hypoxic ischemia coma. JAMA 253:1420, 1985
75. Brain Resuscitation Clinical Trial II Study Group: A randomized clinical study of

calcium entry blocker of lidophlazine in the treatment of comatose survivors of cardiac arrest. N Engl J Med 324:1225, 1991

76. Abramson S, Safar P, Detre K et al: Randomized clinical study of thiopental loading in comatose survivors of cardiac arrest. N Engl J Med 314:397, 1986
77. Winkle RA, Mead HR, Ruder MA et al: Long-term outcome with the automatic implantable cardioverter-defibrillator. J Am Coll Cardiol 13:1353, 1989
78. Weir B: Aneurysms Affecting the Nervous System. Williams & Wilkins, Baltimore, 1987
79. Cooper PR: Head Injury. Williams & Wilkins, Baltimore, 1986
80. Einhaupl KM, Villringer A, Meister W et al: Heparin treatment in sinus thrombosis. Lancet 338:597, 1991
81. Hacke W, Zeumer H, Ferbert A: Intra-arterial thrombolytic therapy improves outcome in patients with acute vertebrobasilar occlusive disease. Stroke 19:1216, 1988
82. Miller JD, Becker DP, Ward JD et al: Significance of intracranial hypertension in severe head injury. J Neurosurg 47:503, 1977
83. Marshall LF, Smith RW, Shapiro HM: The outcome with aggressive treatment in severe head injuries. Part I: the significance of intracranial pressure monitoring. J Neurosurg 50:20, 1979
84. Ott KH, Kase CS, Ojeman RG et al: Cerebellar hemorrhage: diagnosis and treatment. Arch Neurol 31:160, 1974
85. Brott T: Thrombolytic therapy for stroke. Syllabus presented at the Proceedings of American Academy of Neurology Meetings in Boston, Massachusetts, 1991
86. Hauser WA: Status epilepticus: epidemiologic considerations. Neurology 40(suppl.): 9, 1990
87. Busto R, Globus M, Deitrich D et al: Effect of mild hypothermia on ischemia-induced release of neurotransmitters and free fatty acids in rat brain. Stroke 20:904, 1989
88. Sipos E, Kirsch JR, Nauta H et al: Retrograde thrombosis following resection of arterial-venous malformation treated with intra-arterial urokinase. J Neurosurg 76:1004, 1992
89. Hanley DF, Feldman E, Borel CO, Rosenbaum AE: Treatment of sagittal sinus thrombosis associated with cerebral hemorrhage and intracranial hypertension. Stroke 19:903, 1988
90. Newell D, Eskridge J, Mayberg M et al: Angioplasty for the treatment of symptomatic vasospasm following subarachnoid hemorrhage. J Neurosurg 71:654, 1989
91. Higashida RT, Halbach VV, Dormandy B et al: New microballoon device for transluminal angioplasty of intracranial arterial vasospasm. AJNR 11:233, 1990
92. Mohr JP, Kase CS: Cerebral vasospasm. Rev Neurol 139:99, 1983
93. Kassell NF, Torner JC, Haley EC et al: The international study on the timing of aneurysm surgery. J Neurosurg 73:37, 1990
94. Solomon RA, Fink ME, Lennihan L: Early aneurysm surgery and prophylactic hypervolemic hypertensive therapy for the treatment of aneurysmal subarachnoid hemorrhage. Neurosurgery 23:699, 1988
95. Widjicks EFM, Vermeulen M, Hijdra A et al: Hyponatremia and cerebral infarction in patients with ruptured intracranial aneurysms: is fluid restriction harmful? Ann Neurol 17:137, 1985
96. Diringer MN, Wu K, Verbalis J et al: Aggressive fluid administration prevents volume contraction but not hyponatremia following subarachnoid hemorrhage. Ann Neurol 31:543, 1992

97. Allen GS, Ahn HS, Preziosi TJ et al: Cerebral arterial spasms: a controlled trial of nimodipine in patients with subarachnoid hemorrhage. N Engl J Med 308:619, 1983
98. Pickard JD, Murray GD, Illingworth R et al: Effect of oral nimodipine on cerebral infarction and outcome after subarachnoid hemorrhage: British aneurysm nimodipine trial. Br Med J 298:636, 1989
99. Robertson CS, Grossman RG, Goodman RC et al: The predictive pattern of cerebral anaerobic metabolism with cerebral infarction after head injury. J Neurosurg 67:361, 1987
100. Faden AI: Opioid and nonopioid mechanisms may contribute to dynorphin's pathophysiological actions in spinal cord injury. Ann Neurol 27(1):67, 1990
101. Lothman EW: The biochemical basis and pathophysiology of status epilepticus. Neurology 40:13, 1990
102. Treiman D: Treatment of status epilepticus. Neurosci Forum 1(3):11, 1991
103. Kumar A, Bleck T: Intravenous midazolam for the treatment of refractory status epilepticus. Crit Care Med 20:483, 1992
104. Arieff AI, Gauisado R, Lazarowitz VC: Pathophysiology of hyperosmolar states. In Andreoli TE, Grantham JJ, Rector FC(eds): Disturbances in Body Fluid Osmolality. American Physiological Society, Bethesda, MD, 1977
105. Arieff AI, Lach F, Massry SG: Neurological manifestations and morbidity of hyponatremia: correlation with brain water and electrolytes. Medicine 55:121, 1976
106. Sterns RH, Thomas DJ, Herndon RM: Brain dehydration and neurologic deterioration after rapid correction of hyponatremia. Kidney Int 35:69, 1989

5

Spinal Cord Injury

David S. Baskin

The management of the spinal-injured patient poses special challenges from the instant the patient is seen in the field until stabilization hours to weeks later. Even though prehospital trauma care has improved markedly, 29 percent of patients with a spinal cord injury still die before reaching the hospital.[1] Furthermore, in every area of the initial evaluation and treatment, special considerations must be given to the routine resuscitative measures used, or further deterioration in function is likely to occur. Therefore, any trauma victim, particularly one with a head injury who is unconscious and difficult to assess, must be assumed to have a spinal cord injury and treated appropriately until definitive diagnostic studies can be performed to show otherwise.[2]

This chapter discusses management of acute spinal cord injury, considering first the initial evaluation at the scene of the accident and treatment in the emergency department. Initial diagnostic studies and their merits also are discussed. Traction and reduction and other medical management considerations then are reviewed.

EVALUATION AT THE ACCIDENT SCENE

As previously mentioned, a high index of suspicion for spinal cord injury in any trauma victim is crucial. Retrospective analysis has shown that an increased awareness of the need for stabilization prior to mobilization at the scene has been associated with the decline in complete spinal cord lesions by almost 11 percent.[3]

Therefore, if a spinal injury is suspected, immediate neck immobilization is paramount. The usual technique is to pass a firm backboard beneath the victim. After the thoracic spine is immobilized, the cervical spine should be similarly restrained prior to motion. Sandbags are placed alongside the head and neck and secured by 3-in. tape, which is passed from one edge of the backboard across the forehead to the other edge of the backboard. This allows free motion of the jaw and lower face for airway control, while still providing stability surprisingly equal to rigid external orthoses.[2] Soft cervical collars are not valuable, as they do not provide sufficient immobilization.[4,5]

Several other considerations apply, including airway, breathing, and resuscitative efforts. So as to not be redundant, this will be described in the emergency department evaluation.

EVALUATION AND TREATMENT IN THE
EMERGENCY DEPARTMENT

Much like the situation in the field, any patient who arrives at the hospital with a history of trauma, or who is unconscious and cannot give an adequate history, must be assumed to have a spinal injury until proven otherwise. Irreversible spinal cord injury with tragic consequences can occur from even trivial motion of such a patient whose neck has not yet been adequately stabilized. Therefore, if there is *any* chance of a spinal injury, the usual emergency protocol of an ABC (airway, breathing, circulation) survey should be appropriately modified.

As always, evaluation of the airway is the first procedure to perform. However, if the airway is adequate on initial assessment, the patient should be stabilized and left secured "as he or she lies." Oxygen should be administered via face mask or nasal cannula. If the airway is compromised, the first maneuver should be that of the chin lift rather than a jaw thrust or neck extension. This reduces the chance of inadvertent mobilization of an unstable cervical spine injury, which could result in quadriplegia. If simply lifting the chin is not adequate to establish the airway, consideration should then be given to intubation.

Much as one might be inclined to perform a tracheotomy or a cricothyroidotomy, this should be avoided whenever possible. If surgery is required for stabilization of the spine, an anterior operation may be required; with a cricothyroidotomy or tracheotomy in place, the chances for infection increase substantially.

Therefore, intubation is the preferable technique. Nasotracheal intubation is much easier than oral intubation in this setting. This procedure does not require hyperextension of the neck and therefore diminishes the likelihood of aspiration.[6] However, the patient must have spontaneous respirations for this procedure to be successful. If not, laryngoscopically guided oral intubation should be performed gently, with the head and neck immobilized by an assistant. Intubation can almost always be accomplished without neck extension.[2] Tracheotomy or cricothyroidotomy should therefore be reserved for those few cases in which the above is not possible.

Once the airway is cleared and breathing is established, attention should be given to the circulatory status. Hypotension is a significant complication associated with spinal cord injury, and if the neurogenic basis for it is not recognized, inappropriate therapy may be administered. Hypotension associated with spinal cord injury in multiple trauma can be either hypovolemic or cardiogenic in nature or sometimes due to a combination of both.[7] Hypovolemic hypotension can be a sequela of simple hemorrhage, or in many cases the acute spinal injury produces a loss of peripheral sympathetic drive, with a marked decrease in peripheral vascular resistance. This, in turn, produces significant venous pooling in the arms and legs and a decreased cardiac preload.[2]

Initial therapy for hypovolemic shock should include volume expansion and placement of thigh-high compressive stockings or simple wrapping of the legs with elastic bandages to reduce peripheral venous pooling. Intravenous access should be obtained, and administration of isotonic fluid should be initiated. Placing the patient in a Trendelenburg position will increase central venous return and also increase the spinal cord perfusion pressure. Cardiogenic shock, which is usually caused by the loss of sympathetic antagonism of tonic vagal influence, usually presents with bradycardia, despite hypotension. Increasing cardiac filling pressures may not counteract this effect. If volume expansion does not adequately improve the situation, atropine 0.5 to 1.0 mg IV or glycopyrrolate 0.1 mg IV should be administered.[2] If the presumed spinal shock does not respond to the above measures, one should be concerned about either inadequate intravascular volume expansion or intrathoracic or abdominal bleeding that has not been recognized. If the blood pressure remains low, the use of a pressor, such as dopamine or Neo-Synephrine, can be very useful. If no internal bleeding is present, pressors are the mainstay of therapy for spinal shock, as volume expansion alone will not increase the blood pressure because of the loss of peripheral vascular resistance secondary to the loss of sympathetic outflow. Early placement of a central venous line or a Swan-Ganz catheter to monitor cardiac filling pressures is helpful in order to guide therapy. A Foley catheter should be placed both to monitor urine output and to prevent bladder distension. A rapid head-to-toe survey should be performed to establish the presence or absence of other injuries. If the patient is awake and alert, a detailed and careful neurological examination is of paramount importance, both to establish the deficit that is present and to serve as a useful baseline in assessing the success or failure of subsequent interventions. This point cannot be emphasized enough. For example, if a patient is subsequently transported and suddenly reports feeling that function has deteriorated, this is a serious concern—both medially and, much later on, medicolegally. If it turns out that the patient *has* deteriorated, consideration must immediately be given to inadequately treated instability, progressive subluxation in the spine, or other new injury. However, it is entirely possible that the patient is now simply becoming much more *aware* of a deficit, and that indeed no deterioration has actually occurred. For diagnostic, therapeutic, and subsequent medicolegal considerations, there is no substitute for an early careful and thorough neurological examination.

Occasionally, a patient will position his or her head in an unusual and non-neutral position. If the patient is awake and alert and resists reduction of the neck into a neutral position, this should be avoided at all cost. As remarkable as it may seem, an awake and alert patient will always position the neck in a manner that minimizes further damage. Until the nature of the spinal injury and the associated vertebral body disruption is clear, the head should be left in this position.[2]

PHARMACOLOGIC INTERVENTION

Even prior to the initiation of diagnostic radiographs, as soon as a spinal cord injury is even remotely suspected, pharmacotherapy is indicated. After more than 30 years of exhaustive research involving tens of millions of dollars, a landmark study has recently shown that the use of high-dose methylprednisolone is efficacious in the treatment of spinal cord injury.[8,9] The National Acute Spinal Cord Injury Study II compared the effects of high-dose methylprednisolone, naloxone, and placebo in spinal-injured patients. For the first time in the history of spinal cord research, the study clearly documented that the use of high-dose methylprednisolone can reduce the severity and improve functional outcome in human spinal cord injury. The results of this study have produced a new unequivocal standard of care, to the point where successful litigation has arisen from the absence of such intervention.

The study included 387 spinal-injured patients, with injuries most commonly caused by motor vehicle accidents, falls, or water-related injuries. Even patients with "complete" spinal injuries improved after initiation of therapy. Although at times this improvement included recovery of only several adjacent spinal segments, this can be of great significance for a patient who starts out with a spinal level at C5 or C6 and improves to a C7 or T1 level. Patients who were treated 8 hours after injury did not improve and actually did worse than patients treated with placebo.[9] Therefore, administration within an 8-hour window from the time of injury is crucial. Patients should receive a 30-mg/kg IV bolus of methylprednisolone as soon as a spinal injury is suspected. For patients in the field in whom weight estimation is difficult, a 2-g bolus is recommended. Once the loading dose is given, continuous infusion of 5.4 mg/kg/h should be started 1 hour later and continued for 23 hours. The results of treatment after 24 hours are not known and are currently under study. At this point in time, each clinician must decide how best to handle this. As there are deleterious effects of high-dose methylprednisolone over an extended period of time, my practice has been to slowly taper the continuous infusion dosage over 72 hours.

Further research is ongoing to determine how this therapy can be improved. The consensus of opinion is that the primary mechanism of action of methylprednisolone in the spinal-injured patient is by antioxidant protection. More powerful drugs are currently being studied to explore what additional intervention can do in terms of prevention of progressive secondary damage. Methylprednisolone therapy has so rapidly become the standard of care that all future studies can no longer use a control group with no therapy; rather, the control group is now patients treated with the standard methylprednisolone protocol for 24 hours.

RADIOLOGIC EVALUATION

Once the patient has been resuscitated, the airway, breathing, and circulation controlled, and an initial dose of methylprednisolone administered, timely radiologic evaluation is essential to establish definitive therapy. Particularly in the patient with an incomplete spinal cord injury, it is of paramount importance to rapidly diagnose all conditions in which spinal cord compression is present. Several studies have shown that early reduction of the spinal canal back to its normal configuration can significantly improve outcome and even, at times, allow the patient to return to a normal or near-normal state. It cannot be overemphasized that although one certainly wants to take the time required for the initial stabilization and assessment, the evaluation should rapidly proceed to a clear imaging of the spine.

The first step is to obtain a lateral radiograph of the cervical spine. This should be performed with the patient still on the stretcher, all handling of the patient being delayed until the results of the examination are known. Great care must be taken that the lower part of the cervical spine is seen adequately on these films. Superimposition of the shoulders must be overcome. This can usually be achieved by downward traction on the arms. If this is unsuccessful, careful elevation of the arm into the swimmer's position can allow for imaging down to the first thoracic vertebra in almost every case. Tragic consequences caused by inadequate visualization of lower cervical spine are, unfortunately, commonplace. In almost every circumstance, the initial imaging of the lower cervical area has been difficult, and for whatever reason, it is incorrectly and tragically decided that such visualization is not critical.

After it has been ascertained that all seven cervical vertebrae are depicted on the radiograph, the outlines of the bony canal are studied and additional films of the thoracic and lumbar spine in the anterior–posterior and lateral projections are made. An open mouth odontoid view is also part of the initial evaluation, for fracture of the odontoid process may be best seen in this projection. For a suspected cervical spine injury, if anterior-posterior, lateral, and odontoid views are normal, oblique views are obtained. If these show no fracture, computed tomography (CT) scan is the next study of choice.

COMPUTED TOMOGRAPHY

CT has become the mainstay for imaging of spinal injuries (Fig. 5-1). The main advantage of the CT scan is the fact that bone is imaged in exquisite detail. The technique is especially helpful in depicting the size and shape of the bony spinal canal, pedicles, lamina, and spinous processes. The configuration of the canal and the extent of bony encroachment usually becomes immediately obvious. Nonetheless, fractures parallel to the scan plane can be missed, and the spinal canal contents cannot be completely assessed without intrathecal contrast agents. However, opacification of subarachnoid space by intrathecal contrast injection allows for excellent visualization of the spinal cord and nonosseous masses within the canal. Intrathecal contrast enhancement may be performed to augment the CT scan, or the CT scan can follow a conventional radiographic myelogram. In the case of acute spinal cord injury, routine CT without dye is often sufficient to establish a diagnosis, and the injection of dye, usually by lateral C1–C2 puncture with the patient maintained in a stabilized position, can be reserved for those cases in which further delineation of anatomy is required.

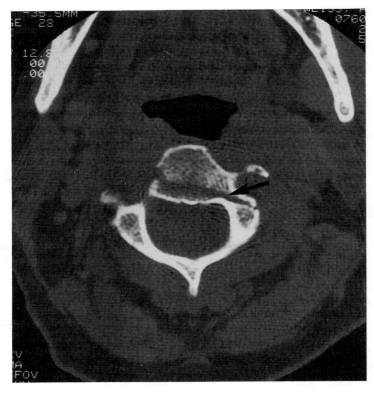

Fig. 5-1 CT scan showing spinal injury. There is an oblique fracture through vertebral body of C2 (arrow). Note exquisite detail of fracture anatomy and close proximity of fracture line to vertebral artery foramen.

Sagittal, coronal, and oblique reconstruction of the spine can usually be performed for demonstrations of fractures in the plane of the section and for evaluation of alignment. The usual protocol for routine examination of the cervical spine consists of a 3-mm slice thickness and 2-mm longitudinal spacing of slices, allowing for a 1-mm overlap. This provides excellent image quality and allows for subsequent reformating. A similar technique can be performed in the thoracic and lumbar spine, in the areas where a fracture is either diagnosed or suspected on the basis of the clinical information and/or plain film imaging. It is usually possible to obtain a detailed understanding of the nature of the bony disruption, which is critical for further treatment.

MAGNETIC RESONANCE IMAGING

Magnetic resonance imaging (MRI) is superior for soft tissue contrast resolution when compared with CT or conventional noninvasive x-ray techniques. Because the spinal cord is well visualized without the use of intrathecal contrast

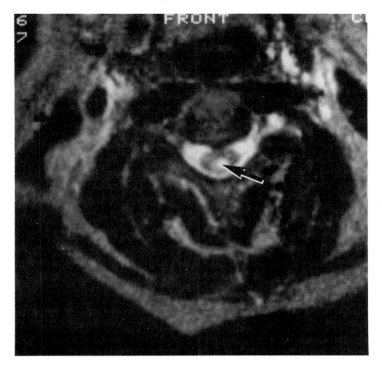

Fig. 5-2 MRI showing spinal injury. This patient became quadriplegic after sudden hyperextension of the neck. No fracture or subluxation was identified. The image shows an area of high signal intensity within the spinal cord, consistent with a cord contusion (arrow).

agents, intra-axial spinal cord lesions are best studied by using MRI (Fig. 5-2). Myelopathy caused by an extra-axial lesion compressing the cord is also well evaluated by MRI, particularly when the process is poorly localized by clinical findings. MRI is particularly useful in the craniocervical junction, where commonly encountered streak artifacts (caused by x-ray beam hardening) seen with CT scan are eliminated. The clear visualization of the medulla and cervical spinal cord is extremely helpful, and the direct sagittal image plane best displays many of the important anatomic relationships in this area. Furthermore, in the case of a normal CT, MRI may demonstrate a significant cord contusion, a hematomyelia, and even a central disc herniation not well visualized by CT. Disadvantages of the study include long examination time. If the patient is to be mobilized with skeletal traction, nonmetallic hardware is essential. The enclosed space often required in most machines also makes it more difficult to manage the patient in the acute setting and presents problems with some patients because of claustrophobia. Nonetheless, if the plain radiographs and the CT scan do not clearly show the nature of the spinal lesion, MRI can be invaluable.

IMMOBILIZATION

Once plain radiographic imaging is obtained, immobilization is essential before patient transfer to CT, MRI, or CT/myelography. In particular, when the cervical spine is involved, immobilization is essential.

In cervical spine fractures, the gold standard technique of initial mobilization is placement of Gardner-Wells tongs (Fig. 5-3). The tongs are placed with the pins just above the pinnae of the ears, on an imaginary plane connecting the mastoid processes and the external auditory canals. Once the tongs have been applied under local anesthesia, traction is initiated in a neutral plane. The initial amount of weight to be applied varies considerably with the level of injury and the amount of suspected disruption of the cervical ligaments. If there is significant ligamentous damage, a minimal amount of weight should be used to avoid distraction and potentially significant neurological deterioration. If there is any uncertainty whatsoever, it is best to start with 5 to 6 lb for upper cervical levels and 10 lb for lower levels and await the initial radiographic evaluation.

After traction is applied, it may well be that additional diagnostic studies are required prior to making therapeutic decisions regarding reduction of the fracture using either open or closed techniques. In such cases, the patient can be transferred to the CT scan in traction, and traction can be maintained throughout the study. If myelography is required, a lateral C1–C2 puncture

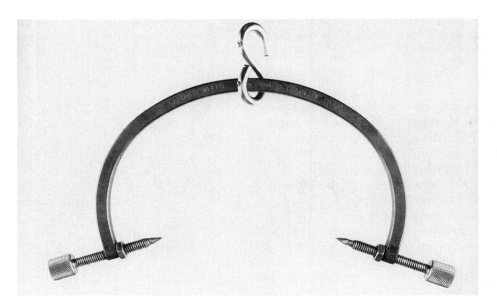

Fig. 5-3 Gardner-Wells tongs. Tongs are easily applied using an injection of local anesthetic and can be used to perform closed reduction of cervical spine injuries, as well as to stabilize an unstable fracture.

can be performed, with the patient's neck immobilized. In the case of MRI, the problem is more difficult, although systems now exist using nonmetallic traction devices.

For thoracic and lumbar fractures, immobilization is more difficult. Although different orthoses do exist, simple bed rest with logrolling of the patient is used initially.

REDUCTION OF SPINAL FRACTURES

Many cervical injuries can be initially treated by closed reduction, using Gardner-Wells tongs and the addition of weights. The initial goal of therapy is to simply restore the alignment of the spinal canal to normal. Injuries such as fracture subluxation without locked facet, unilaterally locked facets, or even occasionally bilaterally locked facets can be initially treated with an attempt at closed reduction. The advantages of such treatment is that a general anesthetic and surgical intervention is avoided during a time of potential instability.

Specific treatment protocols depend on the nature of the injury. For example, hyperextension injuries, where the anterior longitudinal ligament is disrupted, require application of traction posterior to the neutral plane to maintain normal anatomic alignment. Management of unilaterally or bilaterally locked facets may also require posterior or flexion movement of the traction vector.

The use of muscle relaxants is common and useful during such procedures, although one must guard against clouding of the sensorium, and therefore reduction of the ability to perform an adequate neurological examination. Other concerns include respiratory compromise, particularly in high cervical injuries, as well as a sudden reduction in muscle tone that allows overdistraction to occur.

In cervical spine injuries, once the spinal canal integrity has been reestablished and compression of the cord has been relieved, there is no urgency for surgical intervention. Stabilization of the patient's medical status should be achieved while the patient is maintained in Gardner-Wells traction. However, if the patient is stable medically and the fracture is unstable, early surgery for fixation and fusion is indicated to provide for early mobilization. If the patient has a complete spinal injury, there is less urgency for surgery, although the argument concerning early mobilization still holds.

The final decision concerning appropriate treatment will vary, depending on the nature of the injury and the clinical situation. For example, some fractures are best treated with halo immobilization and/or the use of other cervical orthoses; others are best treated with traction, producing closed reduction with subsequent immobilization with bracing; others may require a combination of traction with closed reduction, followed by operative fusion. Early intervention designed at reducing spinal cord compression is paramount (as is detailed diagnostic radiographic imaging) in delineating the exact nature of the disruption, so that appropriate therapy can be instituted.

As far as thoracic and lumbar fractures are concerned, closed traction reduction using halo fixation in the skull with bilateral tibial fixation can sometimes be effective. Surgical intervention may be required, depending on the degree of spinal canal compromise and the nature of the spinal instability that is present.

MEDICAL MANAGEMENT

NURSING CARE

Treatment of the spinal cord-injured patient presents unique challenges because of secondary medical complications related to loss of neurological function. Spinal-injured patients are extremely susceptible to pulmonary, genitourinary, hematologic, and dermatologic, and other complications. From the moment they arrive in the intensive care unit, efforts must focus on preventing these complications, as well as facilitating mobilization and rehabilitation.[10]

CHOICE OF BED

This seemingly trivial consideration can be extremely important. Considerations include the technique for immobilization with traction, as well as prevention of secondary pulmonary and dermatologic complications, and allowing for ease of nursing care. The traditional bed has been the Stryker frame (Stryker Corporation, Kalamazoo, Michigan), which essentially uses a clamshell-type device to immobilize the patient and to turn them either in the prone, supine, or lateral positions. However, advances have been made with beds that are now much more patient- and nurse-friendly, and allow for improved patient stability. The kinetic therapy bed (Rotobed, Rotorest Kinetic Treatment Table, Kinetic Concepts Inc., San Antonio, Texas) is an example of such improvement in technology.[11,12] The Rotobed has been used exclusively in many centers, and its stability and simplicity of use greatly facilitate immobilization, pulmonary care, and basic nursing care.[13–15] Slow rotation is well tolerated by most patients, the arc can be adjusted, and the bed is uniquely designed to allow easy access to different body regions (Fig. 5-4).

PULMONARY CARE

Pulmonary complications are common in patients with spinal cord injuries, particularly in those with injuries to the cervical cord. Problems include mobilization of secretions, adequate lung expansion, avoidance of ventilation perfusion mismatching, and infection. Adequate hydration, incentive spirometry, avoidance of aspiration, and close observation for symptoms and signs of ventilatory compromise or pneumonia must begin immediately. Continuous monitoring of oxygen saturation, using transcutaneous pulse oximetry, has been helpful in this regard, along with frequent changes in position, daily chest radiographs, and careful attention to pulmonary toilet on the part of the nursing staff. Long-term management includes patient and caregiver education concerning the nature of the problems to be expected.

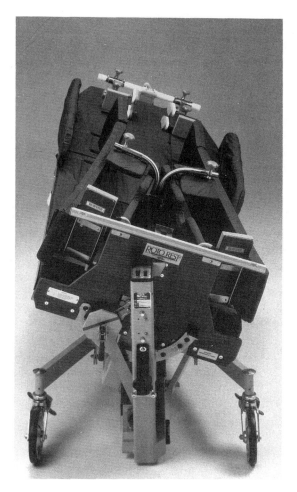

Fig. 5-4 Rotorest bed. Beds such as this have revolutionized care of spinal cord-injured patients. Slow and continuous rotation prevents pressure ulcers and improves pulmonary toilet. Access to various body areas via compartments in the bed has greatly improved ease of nursing care.

DEEP VENOUS THROMBOSIS AND PULMONARY EMBOLISM

Deep venous thrombosis (DVT) and pulmonary embolus (PE) are frequent complications in the spinal cord-injured patient. The first 2 months, and in particular the first 3 weeks, are the most critical.[16] More than 35 percent of deaths within the first 3 weeks of spinal cord injury are due to pulmonary embolus,[17] and the incidence of fatal pulmonary embolism in acutely paraplegic patients is approximately 2 percent. The mortality from pulmonary embolism is highest within the first 10 minutes of the onset of symptoms—roughly

10 percent die within the first hour. The need for rapid diagnosis and treatment is emphasized by the fact that approximately 70 percent of survivors of the first hour are not diagnosed, and 30 percent of these patients will subsequently die. However, mortality can be reduced to less than 10 percent if the diagnosis is made and therapy begun rapidly.

Although DVT of the calves is twice as common as that of the thighs, more than 90 percent of pulmonary emboli are derived from the iliofemoral venous system.[18] After the development of DVT, the risks of fatal PE in all patients is more than 35 percent.[19] Because venous stasis is the most important significant predisposing factor for DVT, spinal cord-injured patients are at high risk, especially if they have other associated risk factors such as age older than 40 years, varicose veins, infection, history of DVT, malignancy, obesity, pregnancy, lupus, or hormonal therapy, including birth control pills.[20]

Because most deaths from pulmonary emboli occur before therapy can be started, prophylaxis is paramount. Pharmacologic rather than mechanical prophylaxis is generally more effective. Leg elevation, physical therapy, and simple elastic stockings do not decrease the incidence of DVT.[21] Although intermittent pneumatic compression and gradient pressure stockings do reduce DVT in paralyzed patients, comparison of this method with low-dose prophylactic heparin has produced variable results.[18,22] Mini-dose heparin prophylaxis (1 unit/k/h of continuous infusion) has proved efficacious in postoperative surgical patients and may be indicated in the high-risk spinal cord-injured patient.[22] Frequent movement of the lower extremities, early physiotherapy, and pneumatic compression stockings can be useful adjuncts. Low-dose intermittent heparin therapy (i.e., 5,000 units administered subcutaneously q 12 h) may also reduce the risk of DVT and PE.

DERMATOLOGIC COMPLICATIONS

A potentially serious complication of immobility after spinal cord injury is the development of the pressure or decubitus ulcer. This complication is particularly devastating in the elderly, who suffer a fourfold greater mortality secondary to pressure ulcers as compared with younger patients.[23] Pressure applied to bony prominences causes a marked decrease in transcutaneous oxygen tension.[24] The sacrum, greater trochanters, ischial tuberosities, lateral malleoli, and heels are the five classic sites for development of pressure ulcers. Prompt treatment is imperative, since sepsis resulting from pressure ulcers in the hospital setting has nearly a 50 percent mortality,[25] and osteomyelitis occurs in nearly 25 percent of nonhealing ulcers.[26]

Prevention remains at the forefront of decubitus management. Animal studies suggest that turning at-risk patients every 2 hours will decrease the incidence,[27] and that alternating supine positioning of the patients with 30 degrees oblique positioning relieves pressure on all five major ulcer sites. Although further studies are needed, early reports show a 50 percent decrease in occurrence of the decubiti in patients when air or water mattresses are used instead of conventional hospital beds.[28] Other methods, including the use of sheepskin mattresses and 2-in. convoluted foam products, appear not to relieve pressure sufficiently. Surprisingly, the popular donut cushion should not be used, as it can lead to ischemia in the center of the donut.[27]

Local ulcer care initially involves removing the pressure sores, along with treatment with topical antibiotics and debridement of the necrotic tissue, using wet-to-dry dressings. Once granulation begins, a moist environment should be maintained. Some advanced ulcers do not respond to medical therapy and may require plastic surgical intervention.

URINARY SYSTEM

Renal failure is the leading cause of death in the chronically spinal-injured patient.[29] One prospective study found that more than 40 percent of deaths were related to kidney disease, which usually manifested as renal failure resulting from a combination of pyelonephritis, hydronephrosis, renal stones, and amyloid.[30] The traumatic interruption of cholinergic innervation of smooth muscle of the bladder, along with adrenergic innervation via the hypogastric nerves and the innervation of the striated external urethral sphincter through the pudendal nerves, affects normal micturation and therefore predisposes to these problems.

The neurogenic bladder may be classified into detrusor hyperreflexia and detrusor areflexia. The former may be further subdivided into hyperreflexia with striated muscle dyssynergia or with smooth muscle dyssynergia. The latter may be divided into areflexia, with nonrelaxing smooth muscle sphincter, denervated striated sphincter,[31] or nonrelaxing striated sphincter. Although the correlation between symptomatology and exact findings on urodynamic testing is poor, consensus indications for urodynamic evaluation include persistently high residual urine volumes on catherization, frequent urosepsis, autonomic hyperreflexia, detrusor hypertrophy, and ureteral dilatation.

Therapy for the neurogenic bladder is aimed at preserving renal tissue by preventing high pressures and infections in the urologic system. During the first stages of areflexia after spinal shock, intermittent bladder catherization has been shown to be the most effective technique.[29] For chronic cases requiring catherization, recent studies have also shown that intermittent catherization is superior to indwelling catheters.[29,32-34] Surgical intervention may be indicated later on in certain spinal cord-injured patients, but there is usually no role for this in early management.

AUTONOMIC DYSFUNCTION

First described in 1917, autonomic hyperreflexia can occur in patients as soon as 2 to 3 weeks after sustaining either complete or incomplete lesions of the cervical or thoracic cord. Massive outflow discharge in the sympathetic nervous system caudal to the spinal cord injury site in response to noxious stimuli results in the signs and symptoms characteristic of this disorder. Nausea, throbbing headache, skin blanching, and diaphoresis below the level of the spinal cord lesion, associated with paroxysmal hypertension resulting from the discharge of uninhibited sympathetic nervous system flow, can produce a frightening clinical picture. Subsequent parasympathetic discharge may cause a reactive sinus bradycardia, as well as nasal congestion and skin blushing above the lesion. Extreme cases may lead to loss of consciousness, seizures, retinal hemorrhage, stroke, subarachnoid hemorrhage, and death.

Although most of the cases of autonomic hyperreflexia occur in patients with a lesion at or cephalad to T5, the disorder has been described in patients with lesions as low as T10.[35–37] Furthermore, 85 percent of patients with lesions above T5, when given the appropriate stimulus, will also exhibit this disorder.[38,39] Virtually any noxious stimulus, including fecal impaction, ingrown toenail, renal colic, manipulation of an indwelling catheter, decubiti, lithotripsy, and urinary tract infection may precipitate the syndrome, though distension of the urinary bladder and uterine contraction are by far the most common causes.[36]

Eliminating the source of noxious stimulation is the primary goal of treatment. In the case of the last two causes mentioned above, use of local epidural or general anesthesia prior to delivery can avert autonomic hyperreflexia, and prompt catheterization of a distended bladder can improve symptoms substantially. At times, additional treatment must be instituted to avert potential life-threatening hypertension. Calcium-channel blockers, such as 10 mg sublingual nifedipine, are effective for prophylaxis and urgent use.[40] Hydralazine and other receptor blockers are not generally considered to be appropriate.[41] In the more severe cases, epidural and spinal anesthesia have been used,[35,36] whereas general anesthesia and potent hypotensive agents, such as nitroprusside and trimethaphan, are used only for the more critical and unresponsive cases.[42]

GASTROINTESTINAL SYSTEM

During the early phases of a spinal cord injury, the insertion of a nasogastric tube using low intermittent suction is indicated to decompress the stomach until gastrointestinal function returns. This minimizes the risks of vomiting and aspiration, with subsequent pulmonary complications. The routine use of H_2-blockers to keep the gastric pH below 5 is recommended.

During the initial period of spinal shock, the spinal cord patient is often incontinent of feces. With the return of the anal reflex, a set routine must be established for patients with lesions above the conus medullaris. A colonic stimulant is usually given several hours before the patient eats. Thirty minutes after eating, suppositories are given, or digital stimulation is begun to induce bowel movement. Conversely, the regular use of bulk agents and enemas for patients with lower motor neuron neurogenic bowel is required, since denervation of the colon and sphincter results in constipation or oozing. This, along with careful regimentation of diet, will greatly facilitate the patient's daily activities.[10]

PHYSICAL THERAPY AND OCCUPATIONAL THERAPY

The early institution of a regular therapy routine is essential in all spinal cord-injured patients. In the incomplete patient, one hopes for a partial return of function over time, and flexibility and function of the muscle groups and joints must be maintained to facilitate rehabilitation. The routine use of range of motion exercise will also reduce the risk of venous thromboembolism and help boost patient morale. Occupational therapy is also of importance in that it gives the patient something to focus on during an extremely traumatic time, when he or she is otherwise left to muse over the devastating aspects of the injury.

PATIENT PSYCHIATRIC CONCERNS

When focusing on the physical aspects of spinal cord injury, one should not forget that, in almost every case, a dramatic change in the patient's life will occur that is likely to be permanent. As in many serious illnesses, patients go through stages of anger, denial, and ultimately acceptance. Immediate attention to this aspect of the injury is critical in order to allow the patient to return to a functional state as early as possible. Rapid involvement of all family members and other patient support systems is extremely helpful, and the use of psychological or psychiatric counseling early in the injury can be beneficial to the patient and the family. Patience and understanding are required from all caregivers. During rehabilitation, whether in an extended care facility, an active rehabilitation program, or at home, consideration must be given to the emotional aspects of recovery if a successful long-term outcome is to be achieved.

ACKNOWLEDGMENT

This work was supported in part by The Henry J.N. Taub Fund for Neurosurgical Research.

REFERENCES

1. Mesard L, Carmody A, Mannarino E et al: Survival after spinal cord trauma: a life table analysis. Arch Neurol 35:78, 1978
2. Chestnut RM, Marshall LF: Early assessment, transport, and management of patients with posttraumatic spinal instability. p. 1. In Cooper PR (ed): Management of Posttraumatic Spinal Instability. American Association of Neurological Surgeons, Parkridge, IL, 1990
3. Gunby P: New focus on spinal cord injury. JAMA 245:1201, 1981
4. White AA, Panjabi MM: Clinical Biomechanics of the Spine. JB Lippincott, Philadelphia, 1978
5. Johnson RM, Hart DL, Simmons EF et al: Cervical orthoses: a study comparing their effectiveness in restricting cervical motion in normal subjects. J Bone Joint Surg Am 59A:332, 1977

6. Sellick BA: Cricoid pressure to control regurgitation of stomach contents during induction of anesthesia. Lancet 2:4046, 1961
7. Meyer GA, Berman IR, Doty DB et al: Hemodynamic responses to acute quadriplegia with or without chest trauma. J Neurosurg 34:168, 1971
8. Bracken MB, Shephard MJ, Collins WF et al: A randomized, controlled trial of methylprednisolone or naloxone in the treatment of acute spinal-cord injury. N Engl J Med 322:1405, 1990
9. Bracken MB, Shephard MJ, Collins WF et al: Methylprednisolone or naloxone treatment after acute spinal cord injury: 1-year follow-up data. J Neurosurg 76:23, 1992
10. Baskin DS, Azordigan P: Non-neurological complications of spinal cord injury. p. 119. In Piepmeier JM (ed): The Outcome Following Traumatic Spinal Cord Injury. Futura Publishing Co., Mt. Kisco, New York, 1992
11. Brackett TO, Condon N: Comparison of the wedge turning frame and kinetic treatment table in the acute care of spinal cord injury patients. Surg Neurol 22:53, 1984
12. McGuire RA, Green BA, Eismont FJ et al: Comparison of stability provided to the unstable spine by the kinetic therapy table and the Stryker frame. Neurosurgery 22(5):842, 1988
13. Green BA, Green KL, Klose KJ: Kinetic therapy for spinal cord injury. Spine 8(7): 722, 1983
14. Gentilello L, Thompson DA, Tonnesen AS et al: Effect of a rotating bed on the incidence of pulmonary complications in critically ill patients. Crit Care Med 16(8):783, 1988
15. Choi SC, Nelson LD: Kinetic therapy in critically ill patients: combined results based on meta-analysis. J Crit Care 7(1):57, 1992
16. Kenasewitz GT, George RB: Management of thromboembolism. Chest 86:106, 1984
17. Guttmann L: Spinal cord injuries: a comprehensive management and research. p. 47. 2nd ed. Blackwell Scientific Publications, Oxford, 1976
18. Broaddus C, Matthay MA: Pulmonary embolism. Postgrad Med 79:333, 1986
19. Stein PD, Willis PW: Diagnosis, prophylaxis, and treatment of acute pulmonary embolism. Arch Intern Med 143:991, 1983
20. Pensak ML, Seiden AM: Postoperative deep venous thrombosis and pulmonary embolism: diagnosis, management, and prevention. Am J Otol 7(5):377, 1986
21. Moser KM, Fedullo PF: Venous thromboembolism: three simple decisions. Chest 83(1):117, 1983
22. Borow M, Goldson HJ: Prevention of postoperative deep venous thrombosis and pulmonary emboli with combined modalities. Am Surg 49:599, 1983
23. Goode PS, Allman RM: The prevention and management of pressure ulcers. Med Clin Am 73(6):1511, 1989
24. Seiler WO, Stahelin HB: Decubitus ulcers: preventive techniques for the elderly patient. Geriatrics 40:53, 1985
25. Bryan CS, Dew CE, Reynolds KL: Bacteremia associated with decubitus ulcers. Arch Intern Med 142:2093, 1983
26. Sugarman B: Pressure sores and underlying bone infection. Arch Intern Med 147:553, 1987
27. Renler JB, Cooney TG: The pressure sore: pathophysiology and principles of management. Ann Intern Med 94:661, 1981
28. Anderson KE, Kvorning JO: Decubitus prophylaxis: a prospective trial of the

efficiency of alternating pressure air-mattresses and water-mattresses. Acta Derm Venereol (Stockh) 63:227, 1982

29. Hackler RH: Urologic care of the spinal cord injured patient. AUA Update Series 3:1, 1984
30. Hackler RH: A 25 year prospective mortality study in the spinal cord injured patient: comparison with long-term living paraplegic. J Urol 117:486, 1977
31. Krane RJ, Siroky MB: Classification of neuro-urologic disorders. p. 150. In Krane RJ, Siroky MD (eds): Clinical Neurology. Little, Brown, & Company, Boston, 1979
32. McGuire EJ, Savastano J: Comparative urological outcome in women with spinal cord injury. J Urol 135:730, 1985
33. Pearman JW: Urological follow-up of 99 spinal cord injured patients initially managed by intermittent catheterization. Br J Urol 48:297, 1976
34. Rhame FS, Perkash L: Urinary tract infections occurring in recent spinal cord patients on intermittent catheterization. J Urol 122:669, 1979
35. Abouleish EI, Hanley ES, Palmer SM: Can epidural fentanyl control autonomic hyperreflexia in a quadriplegic parturient? Anesth Analg 68:523, 1989
36. Ahn JH, Goodgold J: Rehabilitation following central nervous system lesions. p. 4389. In Youmans JR (ed): Neurological Surgery. WB Saunders, Philadelphia, 1990
37. Brian JE, Clark RB, Quirk JG: Autonomic hyperreflexia, cesarean section and anesthesia. J Reprod Med 33:645, 1988
38. Stowe DF, Berstein JS, Madsen KE et al: Autonomic hyperreflexia in spinal cord injured patients during extracorporeal shock wave lithotripsy. Anesth Analg 68:788, 1989
39. Wanner MB, Rageth CJ, Zach GA: Pregnancy and autonomic hyperreflexia in patients with spinal cord lesions. Paraplegia 25:482, 1987
40. Dykstra DD, Sidi AA, Anderson LC: Effects of nifedipine on cystoscopic induced autonomic hyperreflexia in patients with high spinal cord injury. J Urol 138:1155, 1987
41. Lindan R, Leffler EJ, Kedia KR: Comparison of efficacy of α-adrenergic blocker in slow calcium channel blocker in control of autonomic dysreflexia. Paraplegia 23:34, 1985
42. Erickson R: Autonomic hyperreflexia: pathophysiology and medical management. Arch Phys Med Rehabil 61:431, 1980

6

Brain Death and Withdrawal of Life Support

James L. Bernat

The physician caring for a patient with profound and irreversible damage to the cognitive or motor centers of the nervous system may wish to order a treatment plan designed to less than maximally extend the patient's life because of the hopeless prognosis and the known wishes of the patient or family. Such a decision to withhold, withdraw, or limit therapy is among the most difficult decisions that the physician must make, because it runs counter to the usual therapeutic spirit of attempted cure or palliation. In this chapter, I present an approach for such decision making that is ethically and legally sound, and represents the highest standards of medical practice.

I discuss the termination of treatment of four classic neurological syndromes. Brain death and the persistent vegetative state are discussed as prototypes of profound impairments of consciousness. The locked-in syndrome and amyotrophic lateral sclerosis are discussed as prototypes of profound permanent paralysis. The importance of firmly establishing the patient's prognosis before ordering termination of treatment is emphasized, and the ethical and legal implications are addressed. Readers wishing more in-depth analyses can consult the following monographs on the topic as a whole,[1] brain death,[2,3] and the decision to terminate treatment.[4–6]

BRAIN DEATH

Brain death is the colloquial term referring to the determination of human death, using tests that show permanent cessation of functioning of the critical neurons subserving the functions of the cerebral hemispheres, diencephalon, brainstem, and cerebellum. Western society has evolved a consensus that, when the tests for brain death are satisfied, the patient is medically and legally dead, irrespective of continued heartbeat, circulation, cellular metabolism, or other intact somatic physiologic functions. This consensus has permitted the

93

drafting of brain death statutes in most American states and European countries.

Although the conceptual acceptance of brain death has been furthered by the needs for multiorgan transplantation, brain death is not merely a contrivance of neurologists and neurosurgeons to provide a supply of organs for transplant surgeons. There is a philosophic basis for regarding the permanent cessation of brain neuronal functions as the standard of human death.[7] Although there is little controversy remaining in regarding brain death as human death, there remains an active debate on the exact amount of neuronal damage necessary and sufficient for death. This philosophic debate does not alter the clinician's bedside determination of brain death, in which test batteries are standardized and widely accepted.

BEDSIDE TESTS FOR BRAIN DEATH

Brain death is a clinical determination made at the bedside by an experienced clinician, using an accepted test battery. Ordinarily, the determination is made by neurologists, neurosurgeons, anesthesiologists, or intensivists. Algorithms are available for brain death determination for the less experienced clinician.[8] The test battery most widely accepted and commonly used was published in 1981 by the Medical Consultants to the President's Commission for the Study of Ethical Problems in Medicine and Biomedical and Behavioral Research.[9] The tests demonstrate *total* cessation of hemispheric and brainstem neuronal functioning and show *irreversibility* through determining the cause of the brain injury, requiring repeat testing after an interval of time, and excluding potentially reversible causes of brain dysfunction (Table 6-1).

Brain death tests have been thoroughly validated. The tests are delineated conservatively, so there will be no fear of false-positive brain death determination when they are properly applied. There has never been a substantiated report of a patient surviving after satisfying properly conducted and interpreted brain death tests.

Coma and Unresponsivity

Coma and unresponsivity show destruction of the cognitive and motor centers of the brain. The brain-dead patient exhibits the deepest form of coma possible. The patient lies motionless when the ventilator is stopped temporarily. There is no spontaneous movement, no posturing, and no response to noxious stimuli, bright lights, loud noises, or threats to the nasal airway. Reflexes integrated purely at a spinal cord level, such as limb deep tendon reflexes and triple-flexion Babinski signs, may be preserved despite brain death.

The *Lazarus sign* is encountered occasionally during apnea testing. Patients may suddenly elevate both arms and cross them over their chest and touch their chin. This movement is generally believed to result from progressive ischemia of cervical spinal cord motor neurons, producing spontaneous neuronal discharges.[10] It is thus equivalent in implication to intact limb deep

Table 6-1. TESTS TO DETERMINE BRAIN DEATH

I. Proof of Cessation of Whole-Brain Functioning
   A. Coma, unresponsivity
   B. Apnea
   C. Brain stem areflexia
      1. Pupillary reflexes
      2. Corneal reflexes
      3. Oculovestibular reflexes
      4. Gag reflexes
      5. Cough reflexes

II. Proof of Permanence of Cessation of Whole-Brain Functioning
   A. Known pathologic cause sufficient to produce clinical state
   B. Exclusion of potentially reversible causes
      1. CNS depressant drugs
      2. Neuromuscular blocking drugs
      3. Metabolic encephalopathies, including hypothermia, shock
   C. Two examinations separated by time interval

III. Confirmatory Tests
   A. Electrophysiologic
      1. Electroencephalography
      2. Brain stem auditory evoked responses
      3. Somatosensory evoked potentials
   B. Intracranial blood flow
      1. Contrast angiography
      2. Radionuclide angiography
      3. Xenon-enhanced computed tomography
      4. Transcranial Doppler ultrasonography

tendon reflexes: evidence that the spinal cord had not been destroyed from the injury that produced brain death.

Apnea

Apnea shows failure of the medullary breathing centers and is a critical brain death test. Although older sets of brain death tests counted apnea simply as the failure to breathe when disconnected from the ventilator for a few minutes, clearly such a definition is inadequate. The damaged medullary breathing center responds more to a hypercapneic than to a hypoxemic stimulus. The $PaCO_2$ must be permitted to climb to the 50- to 60-mmHg range to maximally stimulate the medullary breathing centers. Without such maximal stimulation, the absence of breathing cannot count as true apnea.

The procedure, permitting the $PaCO_2$ to climb while protecting the PaO_2 from falling to dangerously low levels, is known as *apneic oxygenation.* The patient is ventilated for 30 minutes with 100 percent oxygen ($FiO_2 = 1.0$). The ventilator settings are chosen to permit the $PaCO_2$ to normalize at approximately 40 mmHg from the lower level at which comatose intubated patients are usually maintained. Assuming normal pulmonary function, the PaO_2 should reach at least 300 to 400 mmHg. At this point, the ventilator is stopped and the patient passively oxygenated at 8 to 12 L/min via a cannula, through the endotracheal tube to the level of the carina, or using a T-piece. The $PaCO_2$ rises during apnea at approximately 2.7 to 3.7 mmHg/min.[11]

The duration of apnea is calculated to permit the $PaCO_2$ to reach 50 or 60 mmHg. Beginning at $PaCO_2 = 40$ mmHg, it takes approximately 6 or 7 minutes to achieve $PaCO_2 = 60$ mmHg. The PaO_2 falls during this time but not to dangerously low levels because it began so high. It is unsafe to perform this test if very high PAO_2 levels are unattainable at the beginning of the test or if the patient becomes hypotensive during the test. The pH falls and the blood pressure rises during the apneic period. True apnea is said to be present if there is no respiratory excursion, sighing, hiccuping, or other evidence of spontaneous respiratory functions, given maximal hypercapneic stimulation. Surveys of neurologists and neurosurgeons have shown that most clinicians perform inadequate tests for apnea.

Absent Brainstem Reflexes

All reflexes subserved by cranial nerves and integrated in the brainstem must be absent for brain death. *Pupillary light reflexes* require cranial nerves II and III, the midbrain, and the sympathetic nervous system. They are tested by shining a bright point light source at the pupil and observing for pupilloconstriction. Pupils in brain death are usually midposition in size as the result of sympathetic and parasympathetic denervation. They neither constrict to light nor dilate to dark. Pupillary light reflexes may be affected by medications given during resuscitation or previously ingested by the patient. Widely dilated pupils may result from atropine administration; constricted pupils raise the question of opiate ingestion. The clinician should also consider that the pupils may have been unreactive prior to the brain insult.

Corneal reflexes require cranial nerves V and VII and the pons. They are tested by stroking the cornea with the rolled tip of a cotton-tipped applicator. No direct or consensual blink response should be present in brain death.

Vestibulo-ocular reflexes require cranial nerves III, IV, VI, and VIII and the median longitudinal fasciculus of the pons and midbrain. They are best assessed by observing the response to 30 to 50 ml ice water injected into the external auditory canals (maximal ice water caloric test). Both canals are inspected otoscopically to assure free access to the tympanic membranes. A size-19 butterfly intravenous device is modified by removing the needle and attaching it to a 30- or 50-ml syringe. The patient should be supine, with the head of the bed elevated to 30° above the horizontal. The open tip of the butterfly device is inserted into one external auditory canal until it is a few millimeters from the tympanic membrane. The full ice water contents of the syringe are then delivered into the canal. An assistant is asked to raise the patient's eyelids. The test is performed on the other ear after an interval of a few minutes. Brain-dead patients should have neither reflex movements of the eyes nor any response whatsoever to this test.

Gag and cough reflexes require cranial nerves IX and X and are integrated in the medulla. There should be neither gagging when the pharynx is stimulated with a tongue depressor, nor coughing when the endotracheal tube is irrigated and suctioned.

Exclusions: Drugs, Hypothermia, and Shock

Brain death determination requires proof that a structural lesion is known, sufficient to account for the patient's state, and that reversible causes of global brain dysfunction have been excluded. If a structural lesion is not known and the presence of potentially reversible metabolic or toxic encephalopathies cannot be reasonably excluded, the clinician should delay declaring brain death until the irreversibility of the state can be known with more certainty.

Drugs depressing the central nervous system (CNS) are a common cause of coma in emergency department patients and can mimic the signs of brain death. For example, barbiturate coma can be sufficiently severe to produce coma, apnea, and brainstem areflexia, as well as a flat electroencephalogram (EEG). Neuromuscular blocking drugs can induce a state of profound paralysis and produce apnea and brainstem areflexia.

Several strategies are available if the clinician cannot exclude the effects of CNS-depressing drugs. Serum toxicologic screens can be ordered. The clinician can simply continue to support the patient and wait (hours to days) for depressant drugs to be metabolized, although phenobarbital may persist in toxic concentrations for many days. Confirmatory tests of brain death measuring intracranial blood flow can be conducted. For concern about neuromuscular blocking drugs, if limb deep tendon reflexes are present or if a muscle can be made to contract by electrically stimulating its nerve, these agents are not present in degrees sufficient to interfere with brain death determination.

Severe hypothermia can also mimic brain death, yet produce potentially reversible CNS dysfunction. Brain death protocols require that core temperature exceed 90°F or 32.2°C. When appropriate, hypothermic patients can be rewarmed according to standard protocols. Patients in severe shock should be treated to achieve a systolic blood pressure greater that 90 mmHg before brain death is determined.

Interval Between Examinations

Brain death is usually not determined on the basis of a single examination. At least two examinations are performed, separated by a time interval. If the global brain dysfunction is present on both examinations, it is assumed that it was present as well in the interval separating them. The desired intervals vary as a function of the etiology of brain death and the age of the patient.

Recommended intervals for patients older than 1 year are 24 hours for hypoxic-ischemic damage from cardiac arrest, 12 hours for other known pathogenesis without confirmatory tests, and 6 hours for known pathogenesis with confirmatory tests.

CONFIRMATORY TESTS FOR BRAIN DEATH

Although brain death is primarily a clinical determination, in several instances it is desirable to perform laboratory tests to confirm the diagnosis. Occasionally, the clinical tests cannot be performed safely. Patients with pulmonary edema, adult respiratory distress syndrome, pneumonia, or other causes of pulmonary failure may not be able to have their PaO_2 raised to levels high enough to safely perform the apnea test. Patients with perforated tympanic membranes cannot safely undergo the ice water caloric test for vestibulo-ocular reflexes. Patients with eye damage may not be able to have pupillary, corneal, or vestibulo-ocular reflexes tested accurately.

Another reason for confirmatory tests is to shorten the time interval between tests, to facilitate more expedient organ donation. Finally, it may be desirable in certain cases with medicolegal implications (e.g., homicide) to have "objective" documentation of the brain death determination in addition to the report of the examining physician.

Confirmatory tests are of two types: electrophysiologic and intracranial blood flow. Generally, the electrophysiologic tests are more widely available, easier to perform at the patient's bedside, less invasive, and simpler to interpret. However, they are not as specific for confirming brain death as the tests of intracranial blood flow.

The ideal electrophysiologic test couples the EEG and the brainstem auditory evoked response (BAER). The EEG measures primarily hemispheric cortical activity, whereas the BAER assesses brainstem electrical conduction. The EEG alone is not an ideal confirmatory test because it may be isoelectric (flat) while the brainstem is undamaged. Further, the EEG is more susceptible to metabolic and toxic suppression than the BAER, thus false-positive brain death confirmations with EEG alone will occur more often than with concomitant use of the BAER. Somatosensory evoked potentials show a characteristic pattern in brain death but, if used, should be ordered with EEG and BAER.[12,13]

Tests of global intracranial blood flow (IBF) exploit the fact that there is a total cessation of circulation to the brain at some point in brain death. Several technologies have been developed to measure IBF. Early investigators showed that contrast angiography by catheter instrumentation of the carotid and vertebral arterial systems disclosed absent intracranial blood flow. Later, portable isotope angiography and single photon emission computed tomography with technetium-99m HM-PAO was used less invasively for the same purpose, with a high degree of accuracy.[14] More recently, xenon-enhanced computed tomography (CT) was shown to demonstrate absent regional intracranial blood flow.[15] Most recently, transcranial Doppler (TCD) ultrasonography was shown to have characteristic findings of "reverberating blood flow" in brain death, revealing anterograde blood flow in systole and retrograde flow in diastole.[16] With further development and availability, TCD will likely replace the other tests of IBF because of its ease, noninvasiveness, and accuracy.

BRAIN DEATH IN CHILDREN

The Task Force for the Determination of Brain Death in Children, a consensus panel of representatives from neurology, pediatric neurology, and pediatrics, published their report *Guidelines for the Determination of Brain Death in Children* in 1987.[17] This report has been generally accepted as the standard for pediatric brain death declaration. The only area of serious controversy remaining is the determination of brain death in infants younger than 1 month.

Children older than 1 year are subject to the same rules of brain death determination as adults. All children younger than 1 year must have a confirmatory EEG in addition to the clinical examination findings. Children aged 2 to 12 months require an examination interval of 24 hours regardless of pathogenesis. Similarly, children aged 7 days to 2 months require a 48-hour examination interval. Brain death cannot be declared in children younger than 7 days. Radionuclide angiography confirmatory tests can be performed, which can eliminate the need for the second examination and EEG. The place of the newer confirmatory tests (xenon-enhanced CT and TCD ultrasound) is not agreed upon, because there has been relatively little experience using these tests in infants, and they were also not available at the time of the Task Force report.

BRAIN DEATH AND ORGAN TRANSPLANTATION

The use of brain death declaration is to cease unnecessary, futile treatment and to procure vital organs for transplantation. Brain-dead patients should be considered as candidates for organ procurement. When brain death determination appears imminent following the first examination, the family should be asked if they would consider organ donation. If they wish to further consider donation, the organ transplantation coordinator can be contacted to speak with them. Should they consent to organ donation, the coordinator can ready the procurement team, so that when the patient fulfills the second set of tests and is declared dead, the ventilator can be reattached and the patient moved expeditiously to the surgical suite for organ procurement.

It is standard practice that no member of the organ procurement team participate in the brain death determination and no physician declaring brain death participate in the organ procurement. State and federal regulations are now in place requiring physicians to consider brain-dead patients as potential organ donors and at least inquire from families if they are interested in organ donation. Most families are very interested in organ donation to create some good from an otherwise tragic, meaningless death.

OPPOSITION TO BRAIN DEATH

Occasionally, for religious or emotional reasons, families will indicate that they want all treatments continued despite the declaration of brain death. Physicians faced with this dilemma should attempt to explain to the family that their loved one is dead, and that nothing can possibly bring him or her back to life. If the opposition remains intractable, the compassionate physician should generally continue ventilator treatment and await the inevitable asystole. However, given the "zero" prognosis for recovery, physicians are not obligated to continue other aggressive therapies, such as vasopressor drugs.

The concept of brain death is compatible with the tenets of most believers in Christianity and Judaism. However, some devout Roman Catholics and strict Orthodox Jews, as well as some believers in Eastern religions, reject the conceptual basis of brain death. For these families, it is particularly important to be sensitive to their needs and not insist on brain death determination for their loved ones.

LEGAL ASPECTS

As of November 1991, 44 states in the United States had enacted laws specifically recognizing brain death as a statutory definition of death, and several other states had established high court judicial precedents recognizing brain death as the standard of human death. Only South Dakota has neither type of law. Physicians in South Dakota, however, can comfortably declare brain death when appropriate because it is the medical standard of care in the United States. New Jersey recently enacted a statute prohibiting physicians from declaring brain death in patients for whom the physician is aware that the declaration would violate the patient's "personal religious beliefs."

PERSISTENT VEGETATIVE STATE

More common than brain death and of greater chronicity is the tragic condition known as the persistent vegetative state (PVS). Unlike the brain-dead patient, whose heart will stop beating within a relatively short time irrespective of treatment, the PVS patient can be kept alive for decades with good nursing care. Faced with the PVS patient who will not recover awareness, physicians may desire to or be requested to order a level of treatment that will predictably shorten the patient's life span. Clinicians should be aware of the medical, ethical, and legal aspects of the treatment of such patients and the proper standards of decision making about their care.

Unlike the global neuronal damage in brain death, in PVS neuronal populations of the hemispheric cortices have been diffusely destroyed but the neuronal populations of the brainstem have been largely spared. The most common cause of PVS is a hypoxic-ischemic insult during cardiopulmonary arrest that has preferentially damaged the phylogenetically newer cortical neurons but has preferentially spared the phylogenetically older and more robust brainstem neurons. Other common causes are bilateral hemispheric strokes, advanced Alzheimer's disease, and head trauma.

Patients in persistent vegetative states have retained wakefulness and intact sleep–wake cycles because the ascending reticular activating system of the brainstem remains intact. Despite the wakefulness, however, such patients utterly lack awareness of themselves or their environment because of diffuse damage to hemispheric cortical neurons. Patients in PVS thus have the ironic combination of wakefulness without awareness.

CLINICAL FINDINGS

The fully developed case of PVS has been defined operationally. Patients lie with eyes open when awake and with eyes closed when asleep. When asleep, they can be aroused to wakefulness with verbal or physical stimuli. When awake, however, they are unable to follow commands, engage in sustained visual pursuit, demonstrate any ability to attend to stimuli, or react psychologically or cognitively to visual, auditory, or somasthetic stimuli. Although the question can never be settled with certainty, it is generally agreed that PVS patients cannot think, feel, experience, or suffer.

PVS patients have an absence of purposeful motor activity. Usually they are mute, and language is always absent. They are doubly incontinent and incapable of chewing or swallowing food. They are able to breathe spontaneously and have intact brainstem reflexes. Circulation and blood pressure are maintained. They require gastrostomy tube feedings, and tracheostomy is usually necessary for respiratory care. Because they frequently develop severe contractures, they require daily range of motion physical therapy and attentive skin care.[18,19]

Laboratory studies in PVS achieve only a mild degree of specificity. EEG usually discloses diffuse slow-wave activity and is isoelectric in the most severe cases. Cortical evoked potentials are absent or delayed. Brainstem evoked potentials are normal. Brain imaging studies disclose diffuse damage to both hemispheres, and marked generalized cortical atrophy is seen in long-standing cases. Positron emission tomography scans disclose a reduction in the rate of cortical neuronal glucose metabolism and oxygen consumption to a level similar to that seen in a normal patient in the deepest plane of general anesthesia.

The prognosis in PVS depends on its pathogenesis. Patients have recovered awareness in PVS resulting from head trauma uncomplicated by intracranial hematoma and intracranial hypertension for up to as long as 18 months after injury. PVS from strokes can recover somewhat up to 1 year. PVS from hypoxic-ischemic neuronal damage during cardiac arrest has the worst prognosis. If there is no evidence for recovery of awareness after 1 week, there is approximately a 90 percent chance for no ultimate recovery of awareness. Further durations from hypoxic-ischemic insult and approximate percentages of nonrecovery of awareness are: 2 weeks, 95 percent; 1 month, 99 percent, 3 months, 99.9 percent.[20,21]

DECISIONS TO TERMINATE TREATMENT

Once it is reasonably certain that the patient in PVS will not regain awareness, the physician should attempt to define the appropriate level of treatment. In doing so, physicians need to be knowledgeable about ethical and legal standards of decision making for incompetent, brain-damaged patients. The steps to terminate treatment are outlined in Table 6-2 and enumerated below.

Table 6-2. PROCEDURES TO TERMINATE TREATMENT IN PATIENTS WITH HOPELESS BRAIN DAMAGE

I. Establish Diagnosis with High Degree of Certainty
II. Establish Prognosis with High Degree of Certainty
III. Identify the Patient's Preferences
    A. If competent, discuss them with the patient
        1. Exclude or treat reversible depression
        2. Enhance communication
    B. If incompetent, seek and follow advance directives
        1. Living will
        2. Durable Power of Attorney for Health Care
        3. Valid renditions of patient's wishes by family or friends
    C. If incompetent and no advance directives
        1. Appoint proxy decision maker
        2. With physician, use substituted judgment or best interest standard
IV. Ascertain Family Wishes
    A. If no consensus, try to gain one with family meetings
V. Choose Level of Treatment
    A. If competent, base level of treatment on patient's decision
    B. If incompetent, base level of treatment on joint decision of proxy and physician
VI. Refer to Hospital Ethics Committee
    A. Oversight function to inspect decision-making process
VII. Refer to Court for Judicial Review if
    A. Incompetent, no advance directives, and no proxy
    B. Incompetent, no advance directives, and family disagrees
    C. There is evidence that the proxy has decided nonaltruistically
    D. Recommended by hospital attorney

Ethical Aspects

The ethical concepts of *nonmaleficence* and *respect for autonomy* are relevant here. *Autonomy* refers to the right of patients to be self-governing and to make choices without unreasonable constraints. Because of permanent incompetence, respect for patient autonomy in the context of PVS requires physicians to investigate and follow the previously stated wishes of the patient regarding their present predicament. Many patients have previously executed advance directives instructing their physician and family on a particular course of action should they ever end up in a state of permanent, hopeless unconsciousness.

Advanced directives for health care are of two types. The most popular is the "living will" or written directive, which instructs physicians and families not to institute heroic treatment if the prognosis for recovery is poor. This directive has the advantage of representing the precise wishes of the patient, but is plagued with ambiguity in interpretation. Many living wills use the term *terminally ill*. It may be unclear to physicians whether PVS counts as a terminal illness, since some PVS patients can be kept alive for decades. Similarly, the directive may state that "extraordinary" therapies be withheld to permit the patient to "die naturally." Usually, it is unclear which therapies the patient considers extraordinary, and this interpretation also differs among physicians.

A more flexible advance directive is the Durable Power of Attorney for

Health Care or Health Care Proxy. By this mechanism, a competent patient can appoint another person to have the legal authority to make the patient's health care decisions should the patient be rendered incompetent by illness or injury. A patient should choose this proxy decision maker on the basis of how well the proxy knows the patient's values and to what extent they have the courage to uphold them. The advantage of the proxy mechanism is that it permits greater flexibility: The proxy can adapt the general value system of the patient to make a decision in a particular clinical situation unanticipated by written directives.

Proxy decision makers should attempt to use the standard of *substituted judgment* when deciding for the patient. By this standard, the proxy is asked to reproduce the decision that the patient would have made in the given situation. This choice may or may not be that which the proxy would have chosen.

In a situation in which there are no formal advance directives, the physician should attempt to learn of the patient's preferences by interviewing close family members or friends. Although information obtained by this mechanism is second-hand, and is therefore subject to error and potential conflicts of interest, it should be sought and followed if it appears valid.

When no reliable information can be found about the patient's preferences, the concept of *nonmaleficence* ("do no harm") should be followed. Here a physician can base the decision on their own and the family's perception of the benefits and burdens of treatment. This decision-making mechanism is known as the *best interest* standard. Often, physicians and families will agree that continued treatment of a hopeless PVS will produce emotional and financial burdens unjustified by the benefits of an unconscious existence, followed by an inevitable death. The best interest standard is ethically less powerful than the substituted judgment standard, because it imposes the possibly incompatible value system of someone other than the patient.

Whether hydration and nutrition can be withheld along with medical therapies remains a controversial issue. The answer to this question turns on whether hydration and nutrition count as medical therapies. Ordinary food and water would never be considered a medical therapy for the awake, alert patient. But considering the technologic requirements of a surgically placed gastrostomy tube and an electrical pump to deliver the appropriate amount of nutrition, coupled with the fact that this passively delivered sustenance is often the only factor maintaining life, hydration and nutrition count as medical therapies in the context of the PVS patient, and therefore may be stopped with other medical therapies. The recent U.S. Supreme Court *Cruzan* decision upheld this interpretation, as did the Ethical and Judicial Council of the American Medical Association[21] and the American Academy of Neurology.[22]

Should the decision be made to reduce or withhold treatment, physicians and families can decide jointly on the appropriate level of care. Any or all treatments can be withheld, including resuscitation, ventilators, medications, and hydration and nutrition. Physicians should never withhold basic nursing care designed to maintain comfort, hygiene, and dignity. Orders should be written explicitly, and the basis for these orders should be discussed with nurses and documented carefully in the medical record.

Legal Aspects

In our litigious environment, physicians must be mindful of how the law constrains decision making when withholding or withdrawing treatment. There have been more than 50 high state court judicial decisions and one U.S. Supreme Court decision that have standardized and clarified the lawfulness of decisions to terminate treatment.[23] Also, most states have enacted living will laws or health care proxy laws. Some state have further mandated specific procedures for physicians to follow, such as New York's do-not-resuscitate law. Physicians should understand and follow the laws within their jurisdiction. Hospital attorneys can provide this information.

The issue of physician liability for criminal homicide for allowing PVS patients to die by valid termination of treatment was settled in several high court decisions, most notably *Quinlan* and *Barber*. Physicians who withhold or withdraw treatment to permit such hopelessly ill patients to die are not committing criminal homicide. This finding contrasts with the clear liability for criminal homicide when a physician kills a patient by lethal injection, suffocation, or other *active* means.

The mechanism for decision making and specifying which treatments can be withheld was clarified in several other cases of PVS, particularly *Brophy, Peter, Jobes,* and *Cruzan*. It is clear that patients have the constitutional right to refuse all treatment, including hydration and nutrition and other life-sustaining treatments without which they will die. Physicians are strongly encouraged to seek and follow advance directives executed previously by patients to guide their decisions. States are encouraged to draft legislation designed to encourage patients to make clear their health care preferences in advance. The recently enacted Patient Self-Determination Act of 1990 further requires hospitals receiving Medicare and Medicaid reimbursements to educate patients on the desirability of executing specific advance directives for medical care.

Hospital ethics committees generally should be consulted when *nonterminal* patients are being permitted to die by termination of treatment. The ethics committe provides an oversight role in such cases to protect the interests of the patient. The committee is not authorized to make the decision about the appropriate level of care, a decision that remains in the hands of the attending physician. The committee's function is to inspect the decision-making process to ascertain that (1) the patient's diagnosis and prognosis have been reached carefully; (2) the physician has looked for and followed the patient's advance directives; (3) family input has been considered; and (4) conflicts of interest have been reasonably excluded. This oversight additionally protects physicians by instituting a multidisciplinary approval of the process of their decision making that recapitulates judicial review and renders it unnecessary in most cases.

LOCKED-IN SYNDROME AND AMYOTROPHIC LATERAL SCLEROSIS

Two disorders of the nervous system produce the combination of intact consciousness and intellect with profound paralysis and inability to communicate and manipulate the environment. Physicians may be asked by such patients or their families to withdraw or withhold life-prolonging therapies to permit them to die of their underlying diseases. The considerations for physicians addressing such requests differ from those discussed previously because these patients are mentally competent to consent to or to refuse therapies and are capable of suffering with and without treatment.

CLINICAL FEATURES OF THE LOCKED-IN SYNDROME

The locked-in syndrome was described in 1966 by Plum and Posner as a state of profound de-efferentation produced by a hemorrhage or infarction in the base and tegmentum of the pons. Affected patients remain fully conscious and competent because the lesion does not interfere with the ascending reticular activating system or its projections to the cerebral cortex. Such patients have complete supranuclear paralysis of all limb, trunk, head, and facial movements, except for retained voluntary control of vertical eye and eyelid movements. Often they are mistakenly diagnosed as comatose because of their profound paralysis, pinpoint pupils, absent horizontal vestibulo-ocular reflexes, and other signs suggestive of a massive pontine lesion.

Most locked-in patients die during the acute phase of their illness from progressive brainstem infarction or a complicating illness. A few improve within a few months to make a variable level of recovery. Most of those who survive after 2 months become permanently locked-in. These patients may have intact sensation and are capable of great suffering. Most patients do not require ventilatory support. Communication is particularly frustrating and requires the patient to be taught a code, such as blink once (or look up) for "yes" and blink twice (or look down) for "no." One such patient was reported to have been taught to use Morse Code with his vertical eye movements and dictated a book by this method.

CLINICAL FEATURES OF AMYOTROPHIC LATERAL SCLEROSIS

Amyotrophic lateral sclerosis (ALS) is a progressive degenerative disease of motor neurons of the spinal cord anterior horns, brainstem motor nuclei, and motor cortex. Affected patients develop progressive upper and lower motor neuron paralysis of the limbs, face, larynx, pharynx, trunk, and respiratory muscles. No treatment significantly alters its course, and patients generally die within several months to a few years due to respiratory paralysis or aspiration. When instituted, aggressive intubation and ventilation temporarily prolongs the life of most patients. Consciousness and cognition remain intact, as does sensation, so these patients are capable of suffering.

TERMINATION OF TREATMENT

Occasionally, locked-in patients and ventilator-dependent ALS patients request that their physicians withdraw their treatment and allow them to die. By the ethical concept of respect for autonomy, competent patients have the right to refuse all forms of therapy, including life-prolonging therapy without which they will die. Although it is psychologically difficult for physicians to discontinue life-supporting care for these patients, generally once they have made the choice it should be followed. However, before physicians rush to disconnect them from ventilators or order cessation of their hydration and nutrition, several considerations should be understood.

Physicians should ascertain to the greatest degree possible that the patient's decision has been made after careful, thoughtful, and rational consideration. Wishing to die in such a hopeless situation strikes healthy physicians as a rational choice, but the patient may not have reached this choice rationally. Depression is understandably common in such patients, and after a bad day they may impulsively choose to forego further therapy. Effective communication and careful education and compassionate counseling about their prognosis and condition with and without therapy are essential. Patients should be reassured that their physician will not abandon them and will attempt to keep them comfortable, whichever treatment option they choose. Physicians may regard a decision to abandon further life-sustaining therapy as rational if it has been consistent over time, has the support and encouragement of family members, and if no obvious, potentially reversible depression is present.[24–26]

Patients with ALS need to be educated about the available ventilator options.[27] Ventilator care is not "all-or-none." Patients should be told about the chest shell (Cuirass) ventilator that does not require intubation or tracheostomy and may be able to compensate for nighttime hypoventilation early in the disease course. Similarly, continuous positive airway pressure devices for nose or mouth access may be comfortably worn by patients in early stages of respiratory failure. All ventilators are adaptable for home use, thus ventilator dependency does not necessitate institutionalization. Further, ALS patients need to be educated about cricopharyngeal myotomy and gastrostomy options to compensate for dysphagia.

Effective communication is essential but difficult for this group of patients. Locked-in patients generally can answer only "yes" or "no" by eye movements, and ventilated ALS patients can only mouth words. The effective communication of complex subjects with many nuances, such as decisions to continue further therapy, is categorically limited, thus restricting the extent that families and physicians can be certain of the exact wishes of the patient. This limitation must be acknowledged when attempting to follow the patient's wishes. Physicians and nurses have the duty to enhance communication for these patients to the greatest extent possible.[28]

Comfort care is critical when the ALS patient is extubated or the locked-in patient is removed from hydration and nutrition or other therapies. Once the decision has been made to extubate the ventilator-dependent ALS patient, physicians have the duty to maintain patient comfort during the dying process. Parenteral morphine or benzodiazepines should be administered in dosages sufficient to diminish air hunger or other sources of discomfort in these patients. The possibility that the medication may further speed the patient's demise should not discourage the physician from prescribing adequate dosages of medications to achieve the goal of analgesia and elimination of dyspnea.[29,30–32]

Legal Aspects

Several high court decisions have supported the rights to competent patients with permanently and profoundly paralyzing diseases to refuse life-sustaining therapies, including ventilators and hydration and nutrition. For the locked-in syndrome, the *Putzer* and *Rodas* cases both affirmed the right of locked-in patients to die from refusal of therapy. The courts held that such decisions by competent patients were rational and did not constitute suicide. For ALS patients, the cases of *Perlmutter, Requena,* and *Farrell* similarly upheld the rights of each patient to refuse further mechanical ventilation, thus permitting them to die. The courts held that such decisions were rational and did not constitute suicide and that the patient's tangible interests in avoiding further suffering outweighed any abstract countervailing interest of the state in extending the patients' lives against their wills.

REFERENCES

1. Bernat JL: Ethical issues in neurology. In Joynt RJ (ed): Clinical Neurology. Vol. 1. JB Lippincott, Philadelphia, 1991
2. Pallis C: Brainstem death. In Vinken PJ, Bruyn GW (eds): Handbook of Clinical Neurology. Vol. 57. Elsevier, Amsterdam, 1990
3. President's Commission for the Study of Ethical Problems in Medicine and Biomedical and Behavioral Research: Defining Death: Medical, Legal, and Ethical Issues in the Determination of Death. US Government Printing Office, Washington, DC, 1981
4. Ruark JE, Raffin TA: Initiating and withdrawing life support: principles and practice in adult medicine. N Engl J Med 318:25, 1988
5. President's Commission for the Study of Ethical Problems in Medicine and Biomedical and Behavioral Research: Deciding to Forego Life-Sustaining Treatment: Ethical, Medical and Legal Issues in Treatment Decisions. US Government Printing Office, Washington, DC, 1983
6. Hastings Center: Guidelines on the Termination of Life-Sustaining Treatment and the Care of the Dying. Hastings Center, Briarcliff Manor, NY, 1987
7. Bernat JL: The definition, criterion, and statue of death. Semin Neurol 4:45, 1984
8. Kaufman HH, Lynn J: Brain death. Neurosurgery 19:850, 1986
9. Guidelines for the determination of death: Report of the Medical Consultants on the Diagnosis of Death to the President's Commission for the Study of Ethical Problems in Medicine and Biomedical and Behavioral Research. JAMA 246:2184, 1981

10. Turmel A, Roux A, Bojanowski MW: Spinal man after declaration of brain death. Neurosurgery 28:298, 1991

11. Belsh JM, Blatt R, Schiffman PR: Apnea testing in brain death. Arch Intern Med 146:2385, 1986

12. Daly DD, Pedley TA: Current Practice of Clinical Electroencephalography. 2nd Ed. Raven Press, New York, 1990

13. Chiappa KH: Evoked Potentials in Clinical Medicine. 2nd Ed. Raven Press, New York, 1990

14. Reid RH, Gulenchyn KY, Ballinger JR: Clinical use of technetium-99m HM-PAO for determination of brain death. J Nucl Med 30:1621, 1989

15. Darby JM, Yonas Y, Gur D et al: Xenon-enhanced computed tomography in brain death. Arch Neurol 44:551, 1987

16. Petty GW, Mohr JP, Pedley TA et al: The role of transcranial Doppler in confirming brain death: sensitivity, specificity, and suggestions for performance and interpretation. Neurology 40:300, 1990

17. Task Force for the Determination of Brain Death in Children: Guidelines for the determination of brain death in children. Arch Neurol 44:587, 1987

18. Dougherty JH Jr, Rawlinson DG, Levy DE et al: Hypoxic-ischemic brain injury and the vegetative state: clinical and neuropathologic correlation. Neurology 31:991, 1981

19. Cranford RE: The persistent vegetative state: the medical reality (getting the facts straight). Hastings Center Rep 18(1):27, 1988

20. Levy DE, Coronna JJ, Singer BH et al: Predicting outcome from hypoxic-ischemic coma. JAMA 253:1420, 1985

21. American Medical Association Council on Scientific Affairs and Council on Ethical and Judicial Affairs: Persistent vegetative state and the decision to withdraw or withhold life support. JAMA 263:426, 1990

22. American Academy of Neurology: Position of the American Academy of Neurology on certain aspects of the care and management of the persistent vegetative state patient. Neurology 39:125, 1989

23. Emanuel EJ: A review of the ethical and legal aspects of terminating medical care. Am J Med 84:291, 1988

24. Bernat JL: Ethical issues in the management of amyotrophic lateral sclerosis. In Belsh JM, Schiffman PL (eds): ALS: Diagnosis and Management for the Clinician. Futura, Mt Kisco, NY, (in press)

25. Goldblatt D, Greenlaw J: Starting and stopping the ventilator for patients with amyotrophic lateral sclerosis. Neurol Clin 7:789, 1989

26. Silverstein MD, Stocking CB, Antel JP et al: Amyotrophic lateral sclerosis and life-sustaining therapy: patients' desires for information, participation in decision making, and life-sustaining therapy. Mayo Clin Proc 66:906, 1991

27. Howard RS, Wiles CM, Loh L: Respiratory complications and their management in motor neuron disease. Brain 112:1155, 1989

28. Bernat JL: Ethical considerations in the locked-in syndrome. In Culver CM (ed): Ethics at the Bedside. University Presses of New England, Hanover, NH, 1990

29. Schneiderman LH, Spragg RC: Ethical decisions in discontinuing mechanical ventilation. N Engl J Med 318:984, 1988

30. Smedira NG, Evans BH, Grais LS et al: Withholding and withdrawing life support from the critically ill. N Engl J Med 322:309, 1990

31. American Academy of Neurology Ethics and Humanities Committee (Cranford RE, Beresford HR, Bernat JL et al): Certain aspects of the care and management of profoundly and irreversibly paralyzed patients with retained consciousness and cognition. Neurology 43 (in press), 1993
32. Bernat JL, Cranford RE, Kittredge FI Jr, Rosenberg RN: Competent patients with advanced states of permanent paralysis have the right to forgo life-sustaining therapy. Neurology 43 (in press), 1993

7

Epileptic Emergencies and Status Epilepticus

David M. Treiman

Webster's Third New International Dictionary defines *emergency* as "an unforeseen combination of circumstances or the resulting state that calls for immediate action as . . . a sudden bodily alteration such as is likely to require immediate medical attention."[1] In epilepsy, emergencies consist of acute seizures, serial seizures, or status epilepticus, as indicated in Figure 7-1. The fundamental reason for treating epileptic emergencies is to prevent the development of brain damage from primary factors, such as impaired autoregulation of cerebral blood flow, excessive brain glucose use, or neuronal damage from excitatory amino acid bombardment, or from secondary factors, such as direct brain trauma, lactic acidosis, and hypoxia or hypercarbia.[2]

One of the important considerations in the management of epileptic emergencies is when to intervene with therapeutic agents when a patient is in the midst of an acute seizure. This is determined by how long an acute seizure will last under ordinary circumstances. The best data on the duration of a single seizure have been provided by Bromfield and colleagues.[3] They recorded 123 generalized tonic-clonic seizures on videotape and electroencephalogram (EEG). Some were primarily generalized tonic-clonic seizures, but most were secondarily generalized and were preceded by simple or complex partial seizures. They measured the duration of the generalized tonic-clonic portion of each seizure. The shortest duration of generalized tonic-clonic seizure activity observed by this group was 20 seconds, whereas the longest was 118 seconds. These data suggest that if the generalized tonic-clonic portion of a seizure lasts for more than 2 minutes, it is unlikely to remain a self-limited single seizure, and thus therapeutic intervention should be considered.

Therapeutic intervention for acute seizures takes two forms. First-aid measures are as follows:

1. Clear the area around the patient to minimize possible trauma to the patient.
2. Support the head to prevent bruising.

111

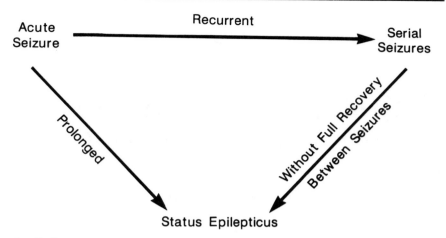

Fig. 7-1 Epileptic emergencies. If a seizure is repeated frequently, such seizures are called *serial seizures*. When the patient fails to fully recover between seizures, this is considered *status epilepticus*. Sometimes a single seizure becomes so prolonged as to appear continuous, and this is also considered to be status epilepticus.

3. Loosen tight clothing, especially at the collar.
4. Turn the patient to the side to avoid aspiration.
5. Do not force an object between the patient's teeth.
6. Do not attempt to restrain the patient.
7. Allow the patient to recover with a minimum of disturbance.

The overall intent of emergency management is to protect the patient from self-inflicted injury to allow the seizure to terminate spontaneously and the patient to recover gradually. These are measures that should be taught to patients' families, teachers, and other individuals likely to render emergency first-aid for seizures. However, if a patient has a seizure within the emergency department or arrives at the emergency department shortly after having had an epileptic seizure, the following procedures should be followed:

1. Establish an intravenous line, using normal saline.
2. Obtain a blood sample for hematology examination and serum chemistries.
3. If there is any suspicion that the patient's seizure may have been due to hypoglycemia, administer 100 mg IV thiamine followed by glucose as 50 ml 50 percent dextrose in water, also intravenously.
4. Evaluate the patient for the cause of the seizures and possible complications (e.g., trauma to the orbital ridge, occiput, spine, or extremities).
5. Determine if the seizure is the patient's first epileptic seizure, is a breakthrough seizure in a patient with epilepsy, or is the first seizure of an episode of recurrent seizures that is going to progress to status epilepticus.
6. Initiate appropriate therapy depending on the results of the evaluation.

If the seizure being evaluated in the emergency department is a breakthrough seizure in a patient with established epilepsy, the patient should be evaluated for the reason the breakthrough seizure occurred. If the patient has been well controlled previously, it is important to ascertain if the seizure occurred because of poor compliance or a transient increase in the metabolism of routine antiepileptic drugs. This information can frequently be obtained by obtaining an accurate history from the patient, friends, or family, as well as by obtaining serum anticonvulsant concentrations. It is also important to determine if the breakthrough seizure occurred as a result of a precipitating event that may have lowered the seizure threshold, such as lack of sleep, severe psychological stress, or alcohol or other recreational drug abuse or withdrawal. Administration of a loading dose of an antiepileptic drug may be necessary to re-establish a serum concentration protective against seizures. The loading dose sufficient to re-establish the desired concentration of an antiepileptic drug can be calculated by determining the difference between the desired antiepileptic drug concentration and the measured concentration and then administering a dose (in mg/kg) equal to the increase in serum concentration desired (in μg/ml). This approximation works because the volume of distribution of most antiepileptic drugs is close to 1 L/kg (Table 7-1) and therefore a 1 mg/kg increase in the dose results in about a 1 μg/ml increase in the serum concentration. The exception to this rule is valproic acid. For this drug, the volume of distribution is approximately 0.25 L/kg, and therefore, a 0.25 mg/kg loading dose will result in a 1 μg/ml acute increase in serum concentration. Caution should be exercised when loading or partially loading patients with most antiepileptic drugs. Large loading doses of carbamazepine, valproate, and primidone may cause gastrointestinal upset, and large loading doses of phenobarbital may cause excessive sedation.

If the serum concentration of the antiepileptic drug is within the therapeutic range or approximates the serum concentration at which a patient has been maintained, there is usually no reason to adjust the dose on an emergency basis.

When evaluating a first seizure, it is necessary to determine whether this is the initial presentation of epilepsy or if the seizure was caused by some other condition. The history is critically important in this determination. A detailed second-by-second description of the seizure should be obtained from both the patient (to the extent that he or she is aware of what happened during the seizure) and from any available observers to classify the seizure properly. It is particularly important to determine whether the seizure began focally or whether the initial behavioral manifestations of the seizure were bilaterally symmetric. Focality of onset implies a cortical localization and, in most cases (with the exception of genetically transmitted rolandic epilepsy and occipital epilepsy in childhood), is a sign of symptomatic or acquired epilepsy secondary to a cortical insult. Seizures of functional etiology (alcohol withdrawal or other metabolic causes) are always bilaterally symmetric in onset, as are most seizures that are manifestations of genetic epilepsies. If a patient with an apparent metabolic or toxic cause for a seizure has focality of onset, this

Table 7-1. DRUGS OF IMPORTANCE IN TREATING STATUS EPILEPTICUS: CLINICAL PARAMETERS AND PHARMACOLOGIC PROPERTIES

	Diazepam	Lorazepam	Phenytoin	Phenobarbital
Intravenous loading dose (mg/kg)	0.15-0.25	0.1	20	20
Maximum rate of administration (mg/min)	5	2	50	100
Effective serum concentration in status epilepticus	200-800 ng/ml	100-200 ng/ml	25-35 μg/ml	20 μg/ml
Time to stop status (min)	1-3	6-10	~10-30	20-30
Effective duration against status	15-30 min	>24 h	>24 h	>24 h
Elimination half-life	30 h	14 h	~24 h	4–6 days
Protein binding (%)	97-99	85-93	87-93	45-50
Volume of distribution (L/kg)	1-2	0.7-1.0	0.5-0.8	0.7
Potential side effects Depression of consciousness	10-30 min	Several h	None	Several days
Respiratory depression	1-5 min	Occasional	Occasional	Consider intubation before administration
Hypotension	Occasional	Occasional	Frequent	Occasional
Cardiac arrhythmias			In patients w/ heart disease	

(Modified from Treiman,[33] with permission.)

suggests the presence of a cortical scar that has been *unmasked* by the metabolic insult rather than *caused* by it.

If there is any suspicion of cortical pathology, the patient should be evaluated for a possible structural lesion with a computed tomography (CT) scan, or preferably magnetic resonance imaging (MRI) study. Even if the description of the seizure suggests bilateral onset of convulsive activity, if the patient has any focality on the neurological examination or the EEG, a possible structural lesion should be considered. Sometimes a partial onset seizure may generalize so rapidly that only the secondarily generalized bilaterally symmetric tonic-clonic seizure activity is perceived by observers.

There has been considerable debate about whether a single seizure should be treated with antiepileptic drugs. Because the definition of epilepsy is a condition characterized by recurrent spontaneous seizures, any patient who has two or more nonprovoked seizures should be treated with antiepileptic drugs. However, many neurologists also initiate antiepileptic drug therapy when a patient has a single seizure and one or more factors on evaluation that predict subsequent seizures. Such factors include focality of onset of the seizure, focality on the neurological examination or EEG or cerebral imaging study, or epileptiform activity on the EEG.

A detailed discussion of choice of antiepileptic drugs is beyond the scope of this chapter, but has been reviewed in several recent publications.[4-6] However, appropriate drugs for a specific seizure type are summarized in Figure 7-2.

As indicated in Figure 7-1, when seizures recur without full recovery of neurological function between them or persist for a sufficient length of time, the patient is considered to be in status epilepticus. For epidemiologic purposes, when seizures occur continuously or more or less repetitively over 30 minutes, such patients are considered to be in status epilepticus. Hauser[7] estimated that approximately 60,000 cases occur in the United States each year. These 60,000 patients can be divided roughly into one-third who have new onset epilepsy, in which status epilepticus is the first presentation of such epileptic seizures, one-third who have established epilepsy or febrile seizures, and one-third in whom status epilepticus is a complication of an acute, severe encephalopathy.

It follows from the definition of status epilepticus that the clinical presentation will depend on the seizure type. The patient may have repeated generalized tonic and/or clonic convulsive seizures in which the patient does not fully recover to a normal level of neurologic function and alertness between the seizures, prolonged attacks of nonconvulsive seizures such as complex partial seizures and absence seizures, in which the clinical presentation is of a prolonged epileptic "twilight" state, or continuous focal seizure activity without any alteration of consciousness. Table 7-2 presents a classification of status epilepticus. By far the most common type of status epilepticus is generalized convulsive status epilepticus. Treiman[8] defined generalized convulsive status epilepticus as paroxysmal or continuous tonic and/or clonic motor activity, which may be symmetric or asymmetric and overt or subtle, but which is associated with a marked impairment of consciousness, especially when convulsions are seen, and with bilateral, although frequently asymmetric, ictal discharges on the EEG. The reason for this broad definition of generalized convulsive status epilepticus is because generalized convulsive status epilepticus represents a dynamic disorder in which the clinical presentation is determined by the stage of status epilepticus in which the patient is first observed. Initially, the patient presents with discrete behavioral and electrographic seizures, each of which has the characteristics of isolated generalized tonic-clonic seizures. However, the longer that generalized convulsive status epilepticus persists without adequate treatment, the more subtle the behavioral manifestations become, so that ultimately the patient exhibits characteristics of what Treiman et al[9] labeled subtle generalized convulsive status epilepticus. In this presentation of generalized convulsive status epilepticus, the patient is almost always in profound stupor or coma and exhibits continuous or intermittent rhythmic subtle motor phenomena, such as eyelid, facial, or jaw twitching, rhythmic nystagmoid eye jerks, or subtle rhythmic focal jerks of the trunk or extremities. The diagnosis of subtle generalized convulsive status epilepticus is made by observing these clinical phenomena in a comatose patient with ictal discharges on the EEG.[10]

Just as there is a progression from overt to increasingly subtle convulsive

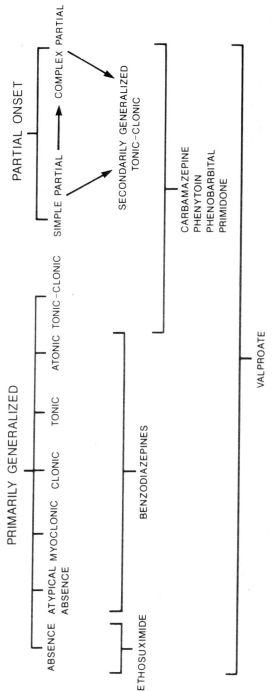

Fig. 7-2 Treatment of seizure types. The International Classification of Epileptic Seizures divides seizures into two fundamental types: those that are generalized from onset (primarily generalized) and those that are partial in onset and may or may not secondarily generalize. Carbamazepine, phenytoin, phenobarbital, and primidone are effective in management of partial seizures and also primarily generalized tonic-clonic seizures. Ethosuximide only prevents absence seizures. Benzodiazepines are occasionally useful in treating some primarily generalized seizure types. Valproate is a broad spectrum antiepileptic drug and may be effective in management of all seizure types.

Table 7-2. CLASSIFICATION OF STATUS EPILEPTICUS

Generalized convulsive status epilepticus (includes both
  primarily and secondarily generalized seizures)
    Overt (generalized tonic-clonic or major motor status
      epilepticus)
    Subtle (most cases of "myoclonic" status epilepticus and
      "electrical" status epilepticus)
Nonconvulsive status epilepticus (epileptic twilight state)
    Complex partial status epilepticus
    Absence status epilepticus (spike-wave stupor)
Simple partial status epilepticus (no impairment of consciousness)

activity during the course of prolonged generalized convulsive status epilepticus, there is also a predictable sequence of progressive EEG changes.[11] Initially, electrographic seizures are discrete and have the EEG characteristics of typical generalized tonic-clonic seizures, which are separated by interictal low-voltage slow activity. As status progresses, these discrete seizures merge together to produce a waxing and waning ictal pattern, which eventually becomes continuous. The continuous seizure activity ultimately is punctuated by periods of relative flattening, which become longer as the ictal discharges become shorter until finally the patient is left with periodic epileptiform discharges on a relatively flat background. This sequence of EEG changes, which was initially recognized in 60 human ictal recordings during generalized convulsive status epilepticus, has been confirmed in six models of experimental status epilepticus in the rat.[11-14] Identification of the EEG patterns that occur in generalized convulsive status epilepticus provides a basis for the diagnosis of generalized convulsive status epilepticus, even when the motor manifestations are extremely subtle. This is important because of increasing recognition that cortical seizure activity may cause profound neuronal damage, even in the absence of convulsive seizures.

TREATMENT

The principles of management of generalized convulsive status epilepticus can be summarized as follows:

1. The longer status persists, the harder it is to control and the more likely that neuronal damage will occur.
2. Neuronal damage is primarily caused by continuous excitatory discharges and not by systemic complications of convulsive activity.
3. However, systemic factors (especially hyperpyrexia) may exacerbate the neuronal damage caused by ictal discharges.
4. Therefore, the goal of treatment of status epilepticus is to terminate all clinical *and* electrical seizure activity as quickly as possible, ideally within 30 minutes.

Several drugs are effective in the management of status epilepticus. Their clinical and pharmacokinetic characteristics are summarized in Table 7-1. However, there are virtually no comparative data that allow the rational choice of one of these drugs over another for the initial treatment of generalized convulsive or any other type of status epilepticus. In six uncontrolled studies,[15–20] phenytoin was effective in 40 percent to 91 percent of patients in status epilepticus. Treiman[21] reviewed in detail the role of benzodiazepines in the management of status epilepticus. In 20 uncontrolled studies, diazepam was effective in stopping different types of status epilepticus in 39 percent to 100 percent of the patients; in nine uncontrolled studies, lorazepam was effective 63 percent to 100 percent of the time.

Only three prospectively randomized comparisons of alternative treatments of status epilepticus have been conducted. Leppik et al[22] found no difference in the efficacy of diazepam versus lorazepam as a first drug in the management of different types of status epilepticus in a double-blind, randomized comparison between these two drugs. In an open but prospectively randomized study, Shaner and colleagues[23] compared the efficacy of phenobarbital and diazepam followed by phenytoin in 36 patients in generalized convulsive status epilepticus, and found no difference in the percentage of patients who responded to these drugs. In the largest comparative trial thus far conducted in the management of generalized convulsive status epilepticus (87 cases), Treiman and colleagues[24] found lorazepam stopped generalized convulsive status epilepticus in 79 percent of the cases when used as a first drug, compared with 49 percent of the cases initially treated with phenytoin.

There remains a need for a large, randomized, double-blind comparison of all the currently popular treatment regimens for generalized convulsive status epilepticus. Such a study is now being conducted in a nationwide Veterans Affairs Cooperative Study involving 15 hospitals.[25] Several protocols[26–30] have been proposed for the management of status epilepticus, and all have merit. Until studies such as the VA Cooperative Study described above are completed, no data exist with which to rationally choose one protocol over another. At the present time, such a choice is best made on the basis of ease of use and experience on the part of the physician with the drugs under consideration. Regardless of the choice of drugs, a prospectively defined protocol for the management of status epilepticus is far more effective than random choice of dose or drugs. Good emergency management requires rapid and vigorous administration of antistatus drugs in doses adequate to stop all clinical and electrical seizure activity. In general, serum concentrations higher than those routinely used for management of chronic epilepsy are necessary to stop ongoing status epilepticus. A protocol for the management of generalized convulsive status epilepticus is provided in Table 7-3. For patients in simple partial status epilepticus—in which, by definition, there is no impairment of consciousness despite ongoing focal seizure activity—high doses of phenytoin should be used to stop the seizure activity, but sedating drugs such as benzodiazepines or phenobarbital should not be used at doses likely to suppress consciousness.

After an episode of status epilepticus has been effectively treated, it is important to support the patient until full consciousness is achieved and to

Table 7-3. TREATMENT PROTOCOL FOR GENERALIZED CONVULSIVE STATUS EPILEPTICUS

1. Make the diagnosis by observing one additional seizure in patient with history of recent seizures or impaired consciousness or by observing continuous seizure activity for more than 10 minutes.

2. Call EEG technician and start EEG as soon as possible, but do not delay treatment while waiting for the EEG unless necessary to verify diagnosis.

3. Establish intravenous catheter with normal saline (dextrose solutions may precipitate phenytoin).

4. Draw blood for serum chemistries, hematology studies, and antiepileptic drug concentrations. If hypoglycemia is suspected, confirm by finger stick. Then administer 100 mg thiamine, followed by 50 ml 50% glucose by direct push into the intravenous line.

5. Administer lorazepam, 0.1 mg/kg by intravenous push (<2 mg/min).

6. If status does not stop, start phenytoin, 20 mg/kg by slow intravenous push (<50 mg/min) directly into intravenous port closest to patient. Monitor blood pressure and electrocardiogram closely during infusion.

7. If status does not stop after 20 mg/kg phenytoin, give an additional 5 mg/kg, and if necessary another 5 mg/kg, to a maximum dose of 30 mg/kg.

8. If status persists, consider intubation before giving phenobarbital, 20 mg/kg, by intravenous push (<100 mg/min).

9. If status persists, start barbiturate coma. Either administer more phenobarbital or give pentobarbital, 5 mg/kg—slowly—as initial intravenous dose to suppress all epileptiform activity. Continue 0.5 to 2 mg/kg/h to maintain EEG suppression. Slow rate of infusion periodically to see if seizures have stopped. Monitor blood pressure, electrocardiogram, and respiratory function closely.

(Modified from Treiman,[10] with permission.)

determine the underlying etiology of the episode of status and correct any precipitating causes for the specific episode.

The prognosis after an episode of generalized convulsive status epilepticus is determined by the rapidity with which status epilepticus is stopped and by the underlying etiology.[31] When status epilepticus is treated rapidly and vigorously, so that all clinical and electrical seizure activity is stopped in the shortest possible time, the outcome is determined by the condition that caused the episode of status epilepticus.[32] However, when treatment is delayed or doses of antiepileptic drugs inadequate to completely stop all seizure activity are used, significant neurological damage or even death may occur in a patient with an otherwise good prognosis. This emphasizes the importance of early, vigorous, and effective pharmacologic management of status epilepticus.

REFERENCES

1. Gove PB: Webster's Third New International Dictionary of the English Language Unabridged. G & C Merriam Co., Springfield, Illinois, 1971

2. Dailey RH: Grand mal (major motor) seizures. p. 292. In Callahan ML (ed): Current Therapy in Emergency Medicine. BC Decker, Philadelphia, 1987

3. Bromfield EB, Porter RJ, Kelley K et al: Progression to generalized tonic-clonic seizures. Epilepsia 30:724, 1989

4. Shorvon S: The treatment of epilepsy by drugs. p. 229. In Hopkins A (ed): Epilepsy. Demos Publications, New York, 1987

5. Mattson RH: Selection of antiepileptic drug therapy. p. 103. In Levy RH, Dreifuss FE, Mattson RH, Meldrum BS (eds): Antiepileptic Drugs. 3rd Ed. Raven Press, New York, 1989

6. Johannessen SI, Loyning Y, Munthe-Kaas AW: The role of antiepileptic drugs in the treatment of epilepsy. p. 505. In Dam M, Gram L (eds): Comprehensive Epileptology. Raven Press, New York, 1991

7. Hauser WA: Status epilepticus: epidemiologic considerations. Neurology 40 (Suppl. 2):9, 1990

8. Treiman DM: Status epilepticus. In Laidlaw J, Richens A, Chadwick D (eds): Textbook of Epilepsy. 4th Ed. Churchill Livingstone, Edinburgh, (in press)

9. Treiman DM, DeGiorgio CM, Salisbury SM, Wickboldt CL: Subtle generalized convulsive status epilepticus. Epilepsia 25:653, 1984

10. Treiman DM: Status epilepticus. p. 183. In Resor SR Jr, Kutt H (eds): The Medical Treatment of Epilepsy. Marcel Dekker, New York, 1992

11. Treiman DM, Walton NY, Kendrick C: A progressive sequence of electroencephalographic changes during generalized convulsive status epilepticus. Epilepsy Res 5:49, 1990

12. Lothman EW, Bertram EH, Bekenstein JW, Perlin JB: Self sustaining limbic status epilepticus induced by "continuous" hippocampal stimulation: electrographic and behavioral characteristics. Epilepsy Res 3:107, 1989

13. Handforth CA, Treiman DM: Electrogenic convulsive status epilepticus—a new model of generalized status. Epilepsia 30:671, 1989

14. Handforth CA, Treiman DM: Increased glucose metabolism associated with "interictal" EEG spiking in the bicuculline methiodine model in rat. Soc Neurosci Abstracts 17:921, 1991

15. Murphy JT, Schwab RS: Diphenylhydantoin (Dilantin) sodium used parenterally in control of convulsions. JAMA 160:385, 1956

16. Carter SH: Use of parenteral diphenylhydantoin (Dilantin) sodium in control of status epilepticus. Arch Neurol Psychiatry 79:136, 1958

17. McWilliams PKA, Leeds MD: IV phenytoin sodium in continuous convulsions in children. Lancet 2:1147, 1958

18. Wallis W, Kutt H, McDowell F: Intravenous diphenylhydantoin in treatment of acute repetitive seizures. Neurology 18:513, 1968

19. Wilder BJ, Ramsay RE, Willmore LJ et al: Efficacy of intravenous phenytoin in the treatment of status epilepticus. Ann Neurol 1:511, 1977

20. Cranford TO, Leppik, JE, Patrick B et al: Intravenous phenytoin: clinical and pharmacokinetic aspects. Neurology 28:874, 1978

21. Treiman DM: Pharmacokinetics and clinical use of benzodiazepines in the management of status epilepticus. Epilepsia 30 (Suppl. 2):4, 1989

22. Leppik IE, Derivan AT, Homan RW et al: Double-blind study of lorazepam and diazepam in status epilepticus. JAMA 249:1452, 1983

23. Shaner DM, McCurdy SA, Herring MO, Gabor AJ: Treatment of status epilepticus: a prospective comparison of diazepam and phenytoin versus phenobarbital and optional phenytoin. Neurology 38:202, 1988

24. Treiman DM, DeGiorgio CM, Kendrick CL, Walton NY: A randomized comparison of intravenous phenytoin and lorazepam in the initial treatment of generalized convulsive status epilepticus. N Eng J Med (submitted)

25. Treiman DM, Meyers PD, Collins JF, Colling C, and the VA Status Epilepticus Cooperative Study Group: Design of a large prospective double-blind trial to

compare intravenous treatments of generalized convulsive status epilepticus. Epilepsia 31:635, 1990

26. Treiman DM, Delgado-Escueta AV: Status epilepticus. p. 53. In Thompson RA, Green JR (eds): Clinical Care of Neurological and Neurosurgical Emergencies. Raven Press, New York, 1980
27. Sutton GG: Emergency management of seizures in adults. p. 165. In Salcman M (ed): Neurologic Emergencies. Raven Press, New York, 1980
28. Delgado-Escueta AV, Wasterlain C, Treiman DM, Porter RJ: Management of status epilepticus. N Engl J Med 306:1337, 1983
29. Hwang PA: Emergency management of seizure disorders. p. 103. In Earnest MP (ed): Neurologic Emergencies. Churchill Livingstone, New York, 1983
30. Treiman DM: Status epilepticus. p. 38. In Johnson RT, (ed): Current Therapy of Neurological Disease. 2nd Ed. BC Decker, Philadelphia, 1987
31. Maytal J, Shinnar S, Moshe SL, Alvarez LA: Low morbidity and mortality of status epilepticus in children. Pediatrics 83:321, 1989
32. Dunn DW: Status epilepticus in children: etiology, clinical features, and outcome. J Child Neurol 3:167, 1988
33. Treiman DM: General principles of treatment: responsive and intractable status epilepticus in adults. p. 377. In Delgado-Escueta AV, Wasterlain CG, Treiman DM, Porter RJ (eds): Advances in Neurology: Status Epilepticus. Vol. 34. Raven Press, New York, 1983

8

Management of Neuromuscular Disease in the Emergency Department and Intensive Care Unit

Sara G. Austin
Karen M. Andrews
Francine J. Vriesendorp

Weakness is the predominant problem in the patient with neuromuscular disease. This weakness can be life-threatening when it involves the bulbar or respiratory muscles. A high level of suspicion is needed in the emergency department so that patients are diagnosed appropriately and rapidly. Particularly meticulous intensive care is warranted, since patients with neuromuscular disease often have an excellent prognosis for complete functional recovery.

The two most common acute neuromuscular problems faced by the evaluating physician are the Guillain-Barré syndrome and myasthenia gravis, which are discussed in this chapter. Other less prevalent neuromuscular problems—such as botulism, acute intermittent porphyria, Lambert-Eaton myasthenic syndrome, tick paralysis, and intoxications causing peripheral nerve disease—have the same basic management, and full discussions can be found in other references. Ventilatory management and general care of the paralyzed patient are common to both diseases and are discussed in the subsequent section.

VENTILATORY FAILURE AND GENERAL INTENSIVE CARE

Ventilatory failure is the most common serious complication in both the Guillain-Barré syndrome and myasthenia gravis. Early recognition and appropriate, prompt action can significantly reduce the associated morbidity and mortality. Most of the recent literature on ventilatory failure has been written on Guillain-Barré syndrome; however, the mechanism (weakness of the respiratory and bulbar musculature) is common to both diseases. Clinical evaluation of the patient with suspected neuromuscular disease must include analysis of respiratory function. A crude but helpful test in the emergency area is to ask the patient to inhale fully and then count quickly from 1 to 25. A patient with adequate ventilatory reserve should be able to do this in one breath. Expiratory forced vital capacity (VC) should be measured at least every 4 hours, more frequently if it is unstable. A baseline arterial blood gas is helpful in the patient with underlying pulmonary disease as well.

Ropper and Kehne[1] recommend that patients be intubated if any of the following criteria are met: (1) mechanical ventilatory failure with reduced expiratory VC of 12 to 15 ml/kg (about 1 L for a 70-kg human), (2) PaO_2 less than 70 mmHg with inspired room air (pulse oximetry is a useful way to follow this), or (3) severe oropharyngeal paresis with difficulty clearing secretions or repeated coughing and aspiration after swallowing. The VC can be difficult to measure accurately secondary to weak facial muscles and poor effort. Care must be taken to seal the lips around the mouth piece and provide encouragement to the patient to make a maximal effort. It is more accurate if serial measurements are made by the same examiner. Vital signs are also useful, with an increasing heart and respiratory rate indicating impending fatigue. Hypercapnia with respiratory acidosis is seen at a VC of 5 ml/kg.[2] One should not wait to intubate until the $PaCO_2$ begins to rise. It is a very late occurrence, and complications such as aspiration pneumonia and hypoxemia from atelectasis are predictable. In our experience, it is wiser to electively intubate in a controlled situation than to try to temporize. In both Guillain-Barré syndrome and myasthenia gravis, respiratory muscle fatigue plays a major role in ventilatory failure. When it occurs, it is not rapidly reversible. Attempting to delay the inevitable is anxiety-provoking for the physician and patient and may be harmful.

Nasotracheal intubation is preferred if there are no contraindications, such as a bleeding disorder. An endotracheal tube with a high-volume, low-pressure cuff should be used, and meticulous respiratory care including chest physiotherapy and frequent cuff pressure measurements are essential. Tracheostomy should be considered if the patient requires ventilatory support for more than 10 to 14 days.

Most intensive care units use volume cycled ventilators, which provide a fixed tidal volume with pressure as the dependent variable. A tidal volume of 12 to 15 ml/kg and an FIO_2 of 25 percent to 30 percent are used initially. The ventilatory rate should be titrated to patient comfort and to maintain a $PaCO_2$

of 35 to 40 mmHg. In the patient without underlying pulmonary pathology who is oxygenating easily, the regular use of a low amount of peak end-expiratory pressure is controversial.

Synchronized intermittent mandatory ventilation (SIMV) is the recommended method of ventilation for most patients with neuromuscular disease. It allows the patient to breathe spontaneously, but supplies a certain, preset number of synchronized breaths per minute. It has the advantage over the assist control method of not allowing the weak patient, who has an increased respiratory rate but low VC, to hyperventilate and develop a respiratory alkalosis.

Weaning is begun as soon as possible. It is accomplished by slowly lowering the SIMV rate. Extubation can be safely performed when the patient can tolerate a T-piece for a preset length of time. Some patients with severe disease are able to tolerate independent breathing during the day; however, they may require assisted ventilation at night for some time.

Patients in the intensive care unit with neuromuscular disease need symptomatic care in addition to specific therapy for their disease. Good nursing care is crucial in preventing the complications of long-term paralysis. Frequent turning to prevent bed sores, psychological support, and meticulous pulmonary toilet are all important. Physical and occupational therapy should be started early to maintain range of motion and provide the patient with tools to increase independence as much as possible. This is most important in the Guillain-Barré patient, who might be paralyzed for months. Physicians must keep constant watch for infection, which is a common complication in Guillain-Barré syndrome and will make a myasthenic patient even weaker. Psychosis may be difficult to recognize in the paralyzed, intubated patient and should be asked about specifically. Patients should be on prophylactic medications for stress ulcers and pulmonary emboli. We use famotidine, 20 mg PO or IV bid, and heparin, 5,000 U SC every 8 hours. Because both Guillain-Barré syndrome and long-term mechanical ventilation predispose to the development of syndrome of inappropriate (secretion of) antidiuretic hormone, serum sodium should be checked routinely.

GUILLAIN-BARRÉ SYNDROME

DIAGNOSIS AND EVALUATION

Guillain-Barré syndrome is a subacute, inflammatory, demyelinating polyneuropathy. The incidence is remarkably uniform and ranges from 0.6 to 1.9 cases per 100,000 population. Epidemiologic studies show that more than 50 percent of patients have had an upper respiratory or gastrointestinal illness caused by viruses or bacteria 1 to 4 weeks before the onset of weakness.[3] Human immunodeficiency virus (HIV) sero-conversion has been associated with the development of Guillain-Barré syndrome.[4] The exact pathogenesis of the segmental peripheral nerve demyelination, which is the hallmark of this disease, is not known, although an immune-mediated mechanism is most likely.

In its milder form, Guillain-Barré syndrome has an excellent prognosis. However, 20 percent to 25 percent of patients require mechanical ventilation, 5 percent to 10 percent have permanent disabling weakness, and 3 percent to 8 percent die from largely avoidable complications, including infection, pulmonary emboli, and cardiovascular instability.[5] Epidemiologic studies have not found a trend in incidence by sex, season, or year.[6] Guillain-Barré syndrome can affect all ages, although it is rare in the very young. Most reports of pediatric Guillain-Barré syndrome have concerned patients older than 2 years. In general, the clinical findings, progression, and outcome have been similar in children and adults. Management and differential diagnosis of pediatric Guillain-Barré syndrome are subtly different, however.[7]

The classic presentation consists of paresthesias beginning in the distal extremities, followed over the next several days by ascending weakness. Examination shows minimal sensory loss, relatively symmetric weakness, and areflexia. Bifacial paralysis is present in one-third to one-half of cases. If severe, the disease progresses to affect the muscles of respiration and deglutition, and autonomic function.[8] More than 90 percent of patients reach their nadir within 4 weeks. A significant proportion of patients present with unusual features, including proximal extremity weakness, monoparesis,[9] bulbar weakness, ataxia and opthalmoparesis (the Fisher syndrome), pandysautonomia,[10] and prominent sensory signs.[11] These disorders are all linked to Guillain-Barré syndrome by similar findings on nerve conduction studies, areflexia, and an elevated spinal fluid protein.[9]

Making a definitive diagnosis in the patient with early disease can be difficult. Laboratory studies, including nerve conduction tests and cerebrospinal fluid examination, are particularly helpful. Nerve conduction studies show multifocal slowing of conduction or conduction block and a predominance of motor fiber involvement over sensory. Absent F-waves, reflecting proximal nerve root involvement, often constitute the earliest abnormal finding. However, nerve conduction studies may be normal initially; therefore, a repeat study in 3 to 7 days is often helpful, as the abnormalities evolve over time. The cerebrospinal fluid classically shows albumino-cytologic dissociation. The white blood cell count is rarely greater than $50/mm^3$ unless HIV infection is present, but the protein is often elevated to more than 55 mg/dl. The abnormally elevated protein, however, may not be present until the second week of the disease.

The differential diagnosis is extensive. In a patient with para- or quadriparesis, it is always most important to make sure there is no evidence of spinal cord dysfunction. Transverse myelitis often presents with similar distal paresthesias and ascending weakness; however, bladder dysfunction is a common and early sign in this disease. Also, spinal shock and a lesion of the corticospinal tracts at the cervicomedullary junction can produce areflexic paralysis, which may be difficult to differentiate from Guillain-Barré syndrome. Table 8-1 lists most of the diseases that can mimic Guillain-Barré syndrome.

The differential diagnosis in children is similar, but also includes infantile botulism and acute cerebellar ataxia. Fortunately, laboratory tests and a careful

Table 8-1. DISEASES THAT MIMIC
GUILLAIN-BARRÉ SYNDROME

Acute transverse myelitis
Diphtheria
Botulism
Carcinomatous meningitis
Periodic paralysis, hypo- or hyperkalemic
Hypermagnesemia
Hypophosphatemia
Tick paralysis
Heavy metal intoxication
Organophosphate poisoning
Acute porphyria
Critical illness polyneuropathy[12]
AIDS-related progressive polyradiculopathy[13]
Polio
Lyme disease
Myasthenia gravis

physical examination can usually differentiate between these. Our usual work-up includes (1) lumbar puncture, (2) nerve conduction studies, including F-waves, (3) urine for porphyria and heavy metal screen, (4) complete blood count and serum chemistries, and (5) HIV and hepatitis serology.

TREATMENT AND PROGNOSIS

All patients with suspected Guillain-Barré syndrome should be hospitalized. The disease is unpredictable and may worsen rapidly. Most patients should be admitted directly to an intensive care unit until it is clear that their disease has stabilized. If a patient has mild disease that, by history, seems to have stabilized by the time the patient presents to the hospital, a regular floor bed with diligent nursing care can be adequate. It should be kept in mind that deterioration may occur at a variable rate over the first 2 weeks of the disease.

Plasmapheresis has been shown by three large randomized controlled studies to be effective in the treatment of Guillain-Barré syndrome.[14–16] It is generally reserved for patients who are unable to walk independently or for those who are able to walk but are continuing to deteriorate over more than 10 to 14 days. It appears to be more effective if instituted within 2 weeks of onset of the disease.[14] A second course of plasmapheresis can be given if there is clear improvement or stabilization lasting more than 1 week, but the patient subsequently deteriorates. In a recent study, 3 of 18 pheresed patients required a second course of plasma exchange.[17]

The regimen we use is a total of 6 treatments performed every other day for 12 days. The rate of exchange is 40 ml/kg per treatment. A continuous-flow machine is used, with albumin and saline as replacement fluids. Serum ionized calcium can be depleted, and we routinely check levels and replace if needed.

Bilateral large-bore antecubital intravenous lines can be used for some patients, but those without adequate peripheral veins should have a double lumen central line placed by someone experienced with their use. We use a Shiley or Quinton catheter for this. Contraindications for plasma exchange are bleeding, hepatic or renal failure, severe electrolyte abnormalities, recent myocardial infarction, or hemodynamic instability. The treatment of children with Guillain-Barré syndrome is no different from that of adults; they, too, benefit from plasma exchange.

The use of steroids has been more controversial. Two randomized, controlled trials of patients with Guillain-Barré syndrome, one using conventional doses of prednisolone for 2 weeks[18] and the other using high-dose intravenous methylprednisolone daily for 5 days,[19] have found no benefit. Therefore, corticosteroids should no longer be considered useful for Guillain-Barré syndrome.

The use of high-dose intravenous immunoglobulin has recently been reported from a Dutch multicenter trial studying 150 patients.[20] Patients were treated who were unable to walk 10 m independently and who entered the study within 2 weeks of onset of their disease. The authors concluded that intravenous immunoglobulin is at least as effective as plasma exchange and may be superior. This result needs confirmation by other controlled trials. Immunoglobulin offers the advantages of ease of administration and universal availability but is very costly. The dose used in the published study is 0.4 g/kg/day for 5 days, infused slowly over 2 to 3 hours. Patients should be excluded from this treatment if they have known selective IgA deficiency or are pregnant. Alternatively, immunoglobulin would be the treatment of choice in the patient with severe Guillain-Barré syndrome who cannot tolerate plasma exchange. The use of immunoglobulin in children with Guillain-Barré syndrome has not been specifically evaluated, however, it has been used safely in children for other diseases.[21] It has a particular advantage in children in whom venous access is often a problem.

Pain can be severe in the patient with Guillain-Barré syndrome and is fairly frequent. It is usually in the low back and proximal muscles. Both tricyclic antidepressants and anticonvulsants have been used with variable results. Positioning can be very helpful, with the knees and hips slightly flexed. Narcotics are frequently necessary, and epidural morphine has been used successfully.[22]

Dysautonomia was found in 65 percent of a large series of patients studied retrospectively at the Massachusetts General Hospital between 1962 and 1981.[23] It is more frequent in those patients with severe motor deficits and respiratory failure. It is manifested as sinus tachycardia, orthostatic hypotension, episodes of bradycardia, heart block and asystole, hypertension, and urinary and gastrointestinal dysfunction. Other causes of tachycardia, hypoxemia, and hypotension must be ruled out such as pulmonary emboli, gastrointestinal bleeding, and fluid and electrolyte disturbances before assuming the patient has autonomic instability. In some cases, the treatments can be worse than the cure, in that these patients can be hypersensitive to drug effects.

Therefore, we treat cautiously with medications that have a short half-life and can be titrated. Esmolol, a very short-acting β-blocker given as a 500-μg/kg/min bolus over 1 minute followed by a maintenance infusion of 25 or 50 μg/kg/min or a nitroprusside drip are both useful to treat severe hypertension and tachycardia. Hypotension can often be adequately treated with the head-down position and intravenous fluid. If needed, low loses of dopamine starting at 2 μg/kg/min can also be used. A rare patient will require a pacemaker. A short period of urinary incontinence is relatively common, being seen in 27 percent of the patients in the series from Massachusetts General Hospital.[24] It can be differentiated from that seen with early spinal cord involvement because it is distinctly uncommon in patients with only mild weakness.

Features shown to have a poor prognosis in studies of patients with Guillain-Barré syndrome are (1) very low distal motor amplitude, (2) older age, (3) ventilatory failure requiring mechanical ventilation, and (4) rapidly progressive disease occurring over 1 week or less. Most patients who are left permanently disabled have required ventilatory support.[25,26]

MYASTHENIA GRAVIS

DIAGNOSIS AND EVALUATION

Myasthenia gravis is the most common disorder of neuromuscular transmission, with an incidence of two to six per million. In adults, it is an acquired disease characterized by formation of antibodies against the postsynaptic acetylcholine receptor (AChR). This causes faulty transmission at the neuromuscular junction by preventing ACh from stimulating the muscle to contract. Myasthenia gravis is a notable exception in the category of neuromuscular disease, as medical and surgical treatment have proven effective both in symptomatic improvement and in altering the natural history of the disease. Despite effective treatment and markedly decreased mortality rates, fluctuations in the severity of the disease often occur unpredictably, and the clinician must be prepared to act quickly when the patient presents with symptoms suggestive of an exacerbation.

Clinically, myasthenia gravis is characterized by fluctuating weakness and fatigability. The weakness may be limited to a few muscles or may be more diffuse. Initially the disease is purely ocular in 40 percent of cases but may generalize. It remains confined to the ocular muscles in only 16 percent of patients. Eighty-seven percent of the generalizations occur within 13 months of onset.[27] Involvement is confined to skeletal muscle, with sparing of autonomic function, sensation, and reflexes.

The diagnosis should be entertained in a patient who shows the characteristic pattern of myasthenic fatigability. A high index of suspicion is needed, since the disease is infrequent and the symptoms can be vague. The diagnosis is corroborated by dramatic improvement following intravenous injection of edrophonium (Tensilon). In an adult, a 2-mg test dose is given; if no severe side effects are noted, such as bradycardia, vomiting, or abdominal cramping, the remaining 8 mg are given. A response should be seen within 30 to 60 seconds. It is important that an objective endpoint, such as improvement of ptosis, ophthalmoplegia, or weakness of a specific muscle group be chosen to minimize the chance of a false-positive result. Because of the possibility of cholinergic complications, atropine must be immediately available. The test should be performed in an intensive care unit setting in patients with known cardiac arrhythmias or who have difficulty managing secretions.

Besides a positive Tensilon test, the diagnosis can be confirmed by a decremental response in the compound muscle action potential on slow repetitive nerve stimulation and a positive antibody titer to the AChR. Because the treatment of myasthenia gravis can include procedures and medications with substantial side effects and, once given, the patient carries the diagnosis for a lifetime, it is mandatory that a definite diagnosis be made and confirmed with objective laboratory tests. The differential diagnosis in the patient with acute or subacute weakness includes peripheral neuropathies such as Guillain-Barré syndrome, botulism, polymyositis, and Lambert-Eaton syndrome. These entities are usually differentiated easily by clinical findings and laboratory studies. Because myasthenia gravis is associated with thyroid dysfunction, other autoimmune diseases and thymic hyperplasia, thyroid function studies, a collagen vascular screen, and a computed tomography or magnetic resonance imaging of the chest should be performed.

Occasionally, the question of myasthenia gravis is raised in a patient who was intubated for another reason but is difficult to wean from the ventilator. The differential diagnosis in these patients includes a defect of the neuromuscular junction similar to myasthenia gravis but caused by drug effect (especially the aminoglycoside antibiotics), critical illness polyneuropathy, and persistent paralysis caused by long-term administration of vecuronium.[28] The evaluation of these difficult patients includes careful repetitive stimulation testing, nerve conduction studies, electromyography, and AChR antibodies.

Myasthenia gravis is a rare condition in children. It can be congenital (onset prior to age 1 year) or acquired. The congenital form has negative AChR antibodies and is caused by a variety of inherited defects in neuromuscular junction transmission. Conventional treatment is not beneficial in these patients.[29] Acquired or juvenile myasthenia gravis has a fairly good prognosis. The etiology is felt to be the same as in adults. A study performed at the Mayo Clinic found that 79 percent of children who underwent thymectomy had remission or improvement. The variables that favorably influenced postoperative remission were early surgery, presence of bulbar symptoms or other immunologic diseases, and onset of symptoms between age 12 and 16 years.[30]

TREATMENT AND PROGNOSIS

Myasthenic patients who come to the emergency department complaining of increasing weakness should almost invariably be admitted to the hospital for observation. The patient with myasthenia gravis can rapidly develop ventilatory inadequacy or bulbar dysfunction with an inability to handle his or her secretions. This may be due to an acute exacerbation of the disease, often caused by underlying infection, thyroid disease, hypokalemia, or administration of a neuromuscular blocking agent. It can also be mimicked by overtreatment with anticholinesterase drugs (cholinergic crisis). In a patient already on Mestinon, the question of myasthenic crisis versus cholinergic crisis can be resolved by performing a Tensilon test. In cholinergic crisis, the patient will become weaker, whereas in myasthenic crisis, improvement is unequivocal. In this situation, controlled ventilation must be instituted, if necessary, before administration of edrophonium.

Pyridostigmine (Mestinon) is the most commonly used anticholinesterase drug. It acts by inhibiting ACh destruction, allowing its accumulation at the synapse. The usual starting dose for a patient who is not in crisis is 60 mg every 4 hours, with frequent evaluations for signs of improvement or side effects. If the patient is unable to take medications by mouth, Mestinon can be given intravenously at a dose of 1/30th of the PO dose. The most common side effect of this drug is autonomic dysfunction, including diarrhea, salivation, lacrimation, increased bronchial secretions, hypotension, and bradycardia. These side effects can be minimized with anticholinergic drugs that act on the parasympathetic nervous system, such as atropine, 0.2 to 0.5 mg. A patient in crisis who has just been intubated rarely responds to pyridostigmine, and it should be held for several days. Patients with purely ocular myasthenia gravis often have a poor response to pyridostigmine as well.

Corticosteroids are effectively used in the treatment of myasthenia gravis. They should be reserved for patients who have significant generalized weakness even after thymectomy or who are unable to tolerate thymectomy. An occasional patient with ocular myasthenia may require steroids if the symptoms are especially disabling and cannot be controlled with other measures such as eye patching and Mestinon. We start or increase prednisone to a high dose, 60 to 100 mg/day, combined with plasma exchange in the patients who are in crisis. This dose of prednisone is maintained for 3 to 6 weeks until the disease has stabilized; then the alternate day dose is tapered slowly. We routinely put patients on prophylactic medications for stress ulcers, usually famotidine, 20 mg PO or IV bid. A low-salt diet with potassium supplementation (20 to 40 mEq/day) is used to diminish fluid overload and the risk of potassium depletion.

Prednisone can transiently exacerbate myasthenia gravis when treatment is initiated or the dose is increased.[31] For this reason, even patients who are not in crisis but who have generalized disease or prominent bulbar symptoms may require hospitalization during the introduction of steroids. Beginning with a smaller dose can decrease the risk of this exacerbation and possibly avoid hospitalization. We commonly use 15 to 20 mg/day to start and then increase slowly.

Patients who do not have an adequate response to steroids or who have unmanageable side effects may require other immunomodulatory drugs. The most commonly used of these are azathioprine[32] and cyclosporine.[33] The disadvantage of these drugs in the intensive care unit setting, however, is that improvement may not be evident for 6 to 24 months.

Plasmapheresis is a valuable adjunct in the treatment of myasthenia gravis.[34] It is reserved for treatment of patients in crisis or in preparation for surgery when steroids are best avoided. The improvement is transient, usually lasting 2 to 4 weeks, and optimum results are attained by using steroids and plasma exchange together when possible. We use the same regimen of plasma exchange for the treatment of myasthenia gravis as is outlined above for the Guillain-Barré syndrome. The contraindications to exchange are also similar.

In most centers, thymectomy is now performed on all adult patients with generalized myasthenia gravis. Individual decisions are made for prepupertal children and the elderly.[27] In a patient with newly diagnosed generalized myasthenia gravis who is a candidate for thymectomy, we use acetylcholinesterase inhibitors and plasmapheresis in preparation for surgery and try to avoid steroids. Postoperative management is usually routine; however, those patients who require a dose of pyridostigmine greater than 750 mg/day, who have had prolonged disease duration greater than 6 years, who have underlying chronic pulmonary disease, or a low VC before surgery have been found to require prolonged postoperative mechanical ventilation.[35,36] These are the same patients who have a poorer prognosis in general.

As a rule, any medication should be used with caution in a patient with generalized myasthenia gravis. Drugs such as curare and succinylcholine, aminoglycosides, quinine and quinidine, β-blockers, and penicillamine are all best avoided, as they can cause myasthenic crisis. The treatment of children with juvenile myasthenia gravis is the same as adults.

REFERENCES

1. Ropper AH, Kehne SM: Guillain-Barré syndrome: management of respiratory failure. Neurology 35:1662, 1985
2. Ropper AH, Kennedy SF: Neurological and Neurosurgical Intensive Care. 2nd Ed. Aspen Publishers, Rockville, MD, 1988
3. Kaplan JE, Schonberger LB, Hurwitz ES et al: Guillain-Barré syndrome in the United States, 1978–1981: additional observations from the national surveillance system. Neurology 33:633, 1983
4. Cornblath D, McArthur F, Kennedy P et al: Inflammatory demyelinating peripheral neuropathies associated with HTLV-III infection. Ann Neurol 21:32, 1987
5. Moore P, James O: Guillain-Barré syndrome: incidence, management and outcome of major complications. Crit Care Med 9:549, 1981
6. Kennedy RH, Danielson MA, Mulder DW et al: Guillain-Barré syndrome. A 42 year epidemiologic and clinical study. Mayo Clin Proc 53:93, 1978
7. Ropper AH, Wijdicks EF, Truax BT: Guillain-Barré syndrome in children. p. 122. In: Guillain-Barré Syndrome. Contemporary Neurology Series 34. FA Davis, Philadelphia, 1991
8. Ropper AH: The Guillain-Barré syndrome. N Engl J Med 326:1130, 1992
9. Koski CL: Guillain-Barré syndrome. Neurol Clin 2:355, 1984

10. Young RR, Asbury AK, Corbett JL, Adams RD: Pure pan-dysautonomia with recovery. Description and discussion of diagnostic criteria. Brain 98:613, 1975

11. Dawson DM, Samuels MA, Morris J: Sensory form of acute polyneuritis. Neurology 38:1728, 1988

12. Bolton CF, Laverty DA, Brown JD et al: Critically ill polyneuropathy. Electrophysiological studies and differentiation from Guillain-Barré syndrome. J Neurol Neurosurg Psych 49:563, 1986

13. Miller RG, Storey JR, Greco CM: Ganciclovir in the treatment of progressive AIDS-related polyradiculopathy. Neurology 40:569, 1990

14. Guillain-Barré Syndrome Study Group: Plasmapheresis and acute Guillain-Barré syndrome. Neurology 35:1096, 1985

15. French Cooperative Group on Plasma Exchange in Guillain-Barré Syndrome: Efficiency of plasma exchange in Guillain-Barré syndrome: role of replacement fluids. Ann Neurol 22:753, 1987

16. Osterman PO, Faguis J, Lundemo G et al: Beneficial effects of plasma exchange in acute inflammatory polyradiculoneuropathy. Lancet 2:1296, 1984

17. Vriesendorp FJ, Mayer RF, Koske CL: Kinetics of anti-peripheral nerve myelin antibody in patients with Guillain-Barré syndrome treated and not treated with plasmapheresis. Arch Neurol 48:858, 1991

18. Hughes RAC, Newsom-Davis JM, Perkin GD et al: Controlled trial of prednisolone in acute polyneuropathy. Lancet 2:730, 1978

19. Hughes RAC: Ineffectiveness of high-dose intravenous methylprednisolone in Guillain-Barré syndrome. Lancet 338:1142, 1991

20. Van der Meche FGA, Schmitz PMI, Dutch Guillain-Barré Study Group: A randomized trial comparing intravenous immune globulin and plasma exchange in Guillain-Barré syndrome. N Engl J Med 326:1123, 1992

21. Lusher JM, Warrier I: Use of intravenous gammaglobulin in children and adolescents with idiopathic thrombocytopenic purpura and other immune thrombocytopenias. Am J Med (Suppl. 4A):10, 1987

22. Rosenfeld B, Borel C, Hanley D: Epidural morphine treatment of pain in Guillain-Barré syndrome. Arch Neurol 43:1194, 1986

23. Truax BT: Autonomic disturbances in the Guillain-Barré syndrome. Semin Neurol 4:462, 1984

24. Ropper AH, Wijdicks EF, Truax BT: Clinical features of the typical syndrome. p. 73. In: Guillain-Barré Syndrome. Contemporary Neurology Series 34. FA Davis, Rockville, MD, 1991

25. McKhann GM, Griffin JW, Cornblath DR et al: Plasmapheresis and Guillain-Barré syndrome: analysis of prognostic factors and the effect of plasmapheresis. Ann Neurol 23:347, 1988

26. Winer JB, Greenwood RJ, Perkin GD et al: Prognosis in Guillain-Barré syndrome. Lancet 1:1202, 1985

27. Engel AG: Myasthenia gravis and myasthenic syndromes. Ann Neurol 16:519, 1984

28. Segredo V, Caldwell JE, Matthay MA et al: Persistent paralysis in critically ill patients after long-term administration of vecuronium. N Engl J Med 327:524, 1992

29. Engel AG, Lambert EH, Mulder DM: Recently recognized congenital myasthenic syndromes: (A) end-plate acetylcholine (ACh) esterase deficiency, (B) putative abnormality of the ACh induced ion channel, (C) putative defect of ACh resynthesis or mobilization. Clinical features, ultrastructure and cytochemistry. Ann N Y Acad Sci 377:614, 1981

30. Rodriguez M, Gomez MR, Howard FM et al: Myasthenia gravis in children: long-term follow-up. Ann Neurol 13:504, 1983
31. Kjaer M: Myasthenia gravis and myasthenic syndromes treated with prednisone. Acta Neurol Scand 47:464, 1971
32. Mertens HG, Reuther P, Ricker K: Effect of immunosuppressive drugs (azathioprine). Ann N Y Acad Sci 377:691, 1982
33. Tindall RSA, Rollins JA, Phillips JT et al: Preliminary results of a double-blind, randomized, placebo-controlled trial of cyclosporine in myasthenia gravis. N Engl J Med 316:719, 1987
34. Keesey J, Buffkin D, Kebo D et al: Plasma exchange alone as therapy for myasthenia gravis. Ann N Y Acad Sci 377:729, 1981
35. Leventhal SR, Orkin FK, Hirsh RA: Prediction of the need for postoperative mechanical ventilation in myasthenia gravis. Anesthesiology 53:26, 1980
36. Eisenkraft JB, Papatestas AE, Kahn CH et al: Predicting the need for postoperative mechanical ventilation in myasthenia gravis. Anesthesiology 65:79, 1986

9

Infections of the
Nervous System

Joseph Berger
Robert M. Levy

This chapter on the critical care of infectious diseases of the central nervous system (CNS) chiefly addresses bacterial meningitis and brain abscess. In the light of the magnitude of human immunodeficiency virus (HIV) infection, the management of acquired immunodeficiency syndrome (AIDS)-related neurological complications is also addressed.

ACUTE BACTERIAL MENINGITIS

PATHOGENESIS

Acute bacterial meningitis is a life-threatening neurological emergency. Mortality rates chiefly are affected by the specific pathogen, the age and underlying medical condition of the host, and the speed with which effective therapy is initiated. With appropriate therapy, current mortality rates generally vary between 5 percent and 30 percent,[1,2] and there appears to have been a perceptible decline in mortality in recent years,[3] with rates as low as 1.5 percent reported in a series from 1982 to 1983.[4] However, under certain circumstances, mortality rates exceeding 50 percent are recorded.[5,6] Logically, the development of sequelae of bacterial meningitis would seem to be largely dependent on factors that influence the mortality rates. Survival and neurological sequelae have been linked to high concentrations of bacteria and bacterial antigen in the cerebrospinal fluid.[7] It is not unexpected that the earlier a diagnosis is established and effective treatment used, the better the chance of survival without neurological sequelae. Curiously, however, despite improvements in the fatality rates of bacterial meningitis with advanced antibiotic regimens, the rate of neurological sequelae does not appear to have changed significantly.[8]

The events leading to neurological sequelae and death in the course of bacterial meningitis are complex, and not likely to be the sole result of exposure to bacterial products. For instance, endotoxin from gram-negative bacteria

135

does not appear to be very toxic to mammalian cells in vitro.[9] The most important events leading to these sequelae are presumed to be the acute meningeal inflammation, with a purulent exudate in the subarachnoid space and the associated elaboration of cytokines.

Leukocytes traverse the blood–brain barrier by unknown mechanisms.[10] The activation of complement by the presence of bacterial antigen, in particular the generation of C5a,[11,12] is chemotactic for neutrophils. Also, the presence of lipopolysaccharides[13,14] and the elaboration of interleukin-1 (IL-1) and tumor necrosis factor (TNF)[13,15,16] increase endothelial cell adhesion for neutrophils, perhaps acting through the up-regulation of different glycoproteins referred to endothelial leukocyte adhesion molecules.[15] The inflammation occurring as a consequence of infection in the subarachnoid space appears to be associated with the production and release of inflammatory cytokines, including IL-1, TNF, and prostaglandins.[10] In experimental studies, the appearance of TNF and IL-1 precede typical cerebrospinal fluid (CSF) changes observed with bacterial meningitis.[17]

The sources of the inflammatory cytokines may include brain endothelial cells[18,19] and resident cells (e.g., microglia/macrophages and astrocytes)[20] (P. Shapsak, personal communication). The generation of these cytokines leads not only to a cascade that results in the elaboration of other cytokines with CNS toxic effects, but also to a neutrophil chemoattraction to the intracranial compartment. A correlation exists between serum TNF levels and fatal outcome in patients with meingococcal meningitis.[21] The initial antibiotic treatment results in the production of large amounts of cytokines in the CSF caused by the rapid lysis of large numbers of bacteria.[9] Corticosteroids may decrease the inflammatory response and limit the neurological sequelae.

The preceding events lead to an increased intracranial pressure, accompanied by an alteration of the blood–brain barrier and cerebral edema, cerebral vascular injury, subdural effusion and empyema, and shock. The consequences of the latter include brain herniation, stroke, seizures, cognitive defects, behavioral disturbances, hearing loss, and visual disturbances. The frequency with which bacterial meningitis results in permanent neurological sequelae varies from 20 percent to 50 percent.[22,23]

The treatment of bacterial meningitis can be divided into several steps including (1) establishing the diagnosis early, (2) using effective antibiotics, and (3) recognizing and treating complications. Reference to recent general reviews[22] on the treatment of bacterial meningitis will cover the first two points in detail.

DIAGNOSIS

Haemophilus influenzae, Streptococcus pneumoniae, and *Neisseria meningitidis* are the microorganisms that most commonly cause bacterial meningitis. The spectrum of organisms responsible for bacterial meningitis, however, is age-dependent. In the neonate, the most common organisms are group B streptococci and gram-negative enterobacteria, particularly, *Escherichia coli.* Meningitis is believed to be more common during the first month of life than at any other 30-day period.[24] In this age group, the illness presents in a nonspecific fashion. A high index of suspicion is required, and lumbar puncture should be performed liberally. In infants and children, the most common causative bacteria is *H. influenzae*, *N. meningitidis*, and *S. pneumoniae* may also be observed. Meningococcal meningitis is seen most often in children and adolescents. Pneumococcal meningitis is typically observed in adults but may be seen at younger ages.

Certain conditions predispose to the development of bacterial meningitis. Penetrating trauma and neurosurgical procedures are associated with staphylococci and gram-negative bacteria meningitis. Pneumococcal meningitis should be considered in the face of sickle cell anemia, alcoholism, and diabetes mellitus. Diabetes also predisposes to infection with gram-negative bacteria and staphylococci. *Listeria monocytogenes* should be considered in the immunosuppressed patient. Although seen with AIDS,[25] it is surprisingly underrepresented in this illness in comparison to its frequency with other causes of cellular immunosuppression.

Clinical features resulting from meningeal inflammation often lead to the consideration of the diagnosis of bacterial meningitis. The patient complains of headache, neck stiffness, and malaise. Seizures and a clouding of consciousness may attend bacterial meningitis. Signs of meningeal irritation are evident, including nuchal rigidity, resistance of movement of the back and legs, Kernig sign, and Brudzinski sign. Kernig sign is characterized by an inability to extend the knee to more than 135 degrees while the hip is flexed.[26] Several signs of meningeal irritation have been ascribed to Brudzinski.[26] Perhaps the most widely recognized is the Brudzinski neck sign, in which passive flexion of the neck is accompanied by flexion of both the thighs and legs.[26] Features of meningeal irritation are not invariably present in the face of meningitis. They are most often absent at the extremes of age. Fever is typically present but may also be absent at extremes of age (the very young or aged patient), in the presence of altered level of consciousness, and in patients with a significant underlying immunosuppression, perhaps as a result of their impaired ability to mount an inflammatory response. A petechial or purpuric rash should suggest the possibility of meningococcal meningitis but may accompany other causes of acute bacterial meningitis. Circulatory collapse may occur in the face of meningococcal meningitis, the Waterhouse-Friderichsen syndrome, and requires the immediate institution of volume expansion, vasopressors, and corticosteroid therapy. Despite the rapid and appropriate medical therapy, it frequently remains fatal.

A lumbar puncture is mandated in the patient with suspected bacterial meningitis. The only absolute contraindication to its performance is the presence of skin or subcutaneous infection in the region through which the needle will pass. The presence of raised intracranial pressure due to an intracranial mass lesion is considered a relative contraindication. In persons with papilledema or focal neurological findings, a computed tomographic (CT) scan of the brain or cranial magnetic resonance image (MRI) may be considered prior to the performance of the lumbar puncture. However, as stated by Fishman,[27] "When there is strong indications for lumbar puncture, such as the need for bacterial cultures if meningitis is suspected, lumbar puncture should be performed despite the possible risks of the procedure." In these instances, a small-gauge (≥22 gauge) needle should be used. The patient should be kept at bedrest after the procedure and carefully monitored. Signs of brain herniation require the immediate institution of appropriate measures for its management (see Ch. 4). Also, a bleeding disorder that cannot be corrected is a relative contraindication to the performance of lumbar puncture.[27]

The opening pressure recorded in the presence of acute bacterial meningitis is typically elevated (>180 mmH$_2$O). A CSF pleocytosis with 1,000 to 10,000 cells/mm^3 is the rule. The cells are predominantly polymorphonuclear. Cell counts greater than 50,000/mm^3 are suggestive of an intraventricular rupture of a brain abscess.[24] Pleocytosis may be absent in rare instances as a result of severe neutropenia. CSF protein levels typically exceed 100 mg/ml, and the glucose is depressed to less than 60 percent of simultaneously recorded serum glucose, but is usually substantially lower with absolute values ≤ 40 mg/ml. In approximately 80 percent of cases of bacterial meningitis, Gram stain of the CSF sediment allows the bacteria to be identified. Counterimmunoelectrophoresis for the presence of bacterial capsular antigens is available for the most common causes of bacterial meningitis, and may provide a diagnosis within 1 hour of the lumbar puncture. Other techniques that may similarly allow for rapid identification of the pathogen include radioimmunoassay, enzyme-linked immunosorbent assay, and latex particle fixation. The value of blood cultures should not be overlooked. Blood cultures often reveal the pathogen for the meningitis; therefore, both the CSF and the blood should be cultured.

MANAGEMENT

Antibiotic Therapy

Selecting the appropriate antibiotic regimen is of critical importance for the appropriate management of bacterial meningitis. For suggested regimens, refer to Table 9-1.

General Management

The presence of dehydration and shock needs to be rapidly assessed in the patient with bacterial meningitis. To rule out the presence of electrolyte abnormalities or a coagulopathy, laboratory studies should include complete blood count with platelet count, prothrombin time, activated partial thromboplastin time, and electrolytes. Dehydration requires volume expansion, and shock may dictate the need for vasopressors.

Petechia and purpura or excessive bleeding after venipuncture suggests the presence of disseminated intravascular coagulopathy (DIC). Treatment of the

Table 9-1. TREATMENT OF BACTERIAL MENINGITIS

Modifying Circumstances	Etiologies	Suggested Regimens	
		Primary	Alternative
Neonate <1 mo	Group B or D streptococci Enterobacteriaceae *Listeria*	Ampicillin + gentamicin or ampicillin + P Ceph 3	Amikacin if gentamicin resistance occurs in 10% or more of isolates in nursery
Infant 1-3 mo	H. influenzae Pneumococci Meningococci + neonatal pathogens	Ampicillin + (cefotaxime or ceftriaxone)	Chloramphenicol gentamicin
Infant >3 mo to child <7 yr	H. influenzae Pneumococci Meningococci	Ceftriaxone or cefotaxime	Ampicillin + chloramphenicol
Child >7 yr Adult 18-50 yr	Meningococci Pneumococci *Listeria monocytogenes*	Penicillin G (HD) or ampicillin (HD) (CSF levels of penicillin higher after bolus than continuous IV [Ann Int Med 112:610, 1990])	Ceftriaxone or cefotaxime or chloramphenicol
>50 yr or alcoholism or debilitating medical condition	Same as adult + Enterobacteriaceae, H. influenzae (rare; *Pseudomonas* sp.)	(Penicillin G [HD] or ampicillin [HD]) + (ceftriaxone or cefotaxime) (If gram-positive diplococci on Gram stain of CSF, penicillin G [HD] adequate)	Aztreonam + TMP/ SMX
HIV-1 infected (AIDS)	+ Cryptococcus neoformans	Amphotericin B (0.5-0.7 mg/kg/day) Fluconazole (400 mg/day) as initial treatment, then 100-200 mg/ day maintenance	
Postneurosurgical procedure or post–cranial spinal trauma	*Staphylococcus aureus* Enterobacteriaceae *Pseudomonas* sp. Pneumococci	Vancomycin + ceftazidime	
Persistent CSF leak	Pneumococci	Penicillin G (HD)	Ceftriaxone or chloramphenicol
Ventriculoperitoneal or other CNS shunt	*Staphylococcus epidermidis* Diptheroids Enterobacteriaceae (rare)	Vancomycin + rifampin (P Ceph 3 if GNB on Gram stain of CSF)	

Abbreviations: P Ceph 3, parenteral third-generation cephalosporin; TMP/SMX, Trimethoprim/sulfamethoxazole; GNB, Gram negative bacteria.
(Adapted from Sanford,[99] with permission.)

underlying abnormality is the more rewarding strategy for the management of DIC; however, intravenous heparin administration should be considered.

Cerebral Edema

As stated, an elevated opening pressure is the rule with bacterial meningitis. CSF pressures in excess of 400 mmH$_2$O suggest a significant associated brain swelling. The mechanism of cerebral edema in the face of bacterial meningitis includes an alteration of the blood–brain barrier resulting from toxins or other substances of the encapsulated bacteria.[28,29] Significant cerebral edema is usually associated with high CSF bacteria counts. Edema may occur in the face of severe neutropenia, indicating that the polymorphonuclear cell is not essential to its development. Other mechanisms for the genesis of cerebral edema with bacterial meningitis include (1) cytotoxic edema; (2) impaired CSF absorption; (3) blockage of CSF paths; (4) cortical vein or venous sinus thrombosis; and (5) fluid overload secondary to the syndrome of inappropriate antidiuretic hormone or iatrogenic etiology.[30]

Clinical features of increased intracranial pressure include a depressed level of consciousness, severe headache, projectile vomiting, depressed pulse and elevated blood pressure (Kocher-Cushing reflex), papilledema, and posturing. Radiographic imaging may indicate brain swelling, and is also essential to determine the presence of associated mass lesions that may contribute to the elevation in CSF pressure. The initial management of increased intracranial pressure is intubation and controlled hyperventilation to lower PCO$_2$ to 25 mmHg. Osmotic agents, such as glycerol or mannitol, should be added to the treatment regimen. The use of corticosteroids, such as dexamethasone 4 to 6 mg IV every 4 to 6 hours, should also be considered.

Hydrocephalus may also complicate bacterial meningitis. Noncommunicating hydrocephalus may occur as a result of a blockage of the aqueduct of Sylvius or the egress from the fourth ventricle. Noncommunicating hydrocephalus may be a neurosurgical emergency. Communicating hydrocephalus may occur as a consequence of impaired absorptive mechanisms of the pacchionian villi.

Seizures

The pathogenesis of seizures in bacterial meningitis includes fever (particularly in children), electrolyte abnormalities, cerebritis, brain abscess, and brain infarction, which may be the consequence of either an arteritis or cortical thrombophlebitis. Management is essentially no different than for seizures that occur in other contexts. Diazepam or lorazepam should be the initial therapy, and a longer-acting anticonvulsant, such as phenytoin, should be started as well.

The routine use of corticosteroids in the management of acute bacterial meningitis remains controversial. Despite the absence of supporting hard data, the accepted standard of care of patients with impending brain herniation as a result of bacterial meningitis is the administration of corticosteroids.

There is also a significant theoretic rationale for the use of corticosteroids and nonsteroidal inflammatory agents to mitigate the consequences of inflammation in the presence of bacterial meningitis.[18,31] Corticosteroids have been shown to decrease the morbidity and mortality of tuberculous meningitis,[32] its salutory effect has been related to the effect on cerebral edema.[33] Corticosteroid administration in children with bacterial meningitis administered during the first 4 days of infection substantially reduce the risk of deafness in children with *H. influenzae*.[34] Similarly, another study in infants and children with bacterial meningitis showed that the administration of dexamethasone before the administration of antibiotics resulted in a significant beneficial effect, including a decrease in the CSF concentrations of TNF-α and platelet activating factor.[35] Also, the clinical condition and the subsequent neurological and audiologic complications in the treated group were significantly improved compared with the group not receiving dexamethasone.[35] The authors[35] suggested that the pernicious effects of endotoxins released by the rapid lysis of microorganisms within the CSF because of the administration of antibiotics could be mollified by the early administration of dexamethasone.

BRAIN ABSCESS

PATHOGENESIS

Brain abscesses develop when microorganisms seed necrotic areas of the brain parenchyma. The development of brain abscesses after parenchymal inoculation has been investigated in a canine model of streptococcal abscess.[36] Four histopathologic stages of abscess formation have been characterized. The early cerebritis stage (days 1 to 3 after inoculation) is characterized by a central necrosis and local perivascular inflammation with associated edema. At this point, the infection is not well demarcated from the surrounding brain. In the late cerebritis stage (days 4 to 9), pus develops and enlarges the necrotic center, around which is a zone of macrophages and inflammatory cells. A reticulin network is deposited by fibroblasts; this is a precursor of the collagen abscess capsule. The early encapsulation stage follows (days 10 to 13), during which the capsule matures. The abscess capsule limits the spread of infection and associated destruction of the brain parenchyma. Because of the relatively lesser vascularity of the deep white matter, the abscess capsule develops more slowly and less completely on the medial side of the abscess. By the late capsule stage (day 14 and onward), the abscess is characterized by five histologic zones: the necrotic center, a peripheral zone of inflammatory cells and fibroblasts, the abscess capsule, a zone of neovascularity and cerebritis, and the surrounding area of edema and reactive gliosis.

The microorganisms causing brain abscesses enter the brain by trauma, by the direct extension of local infection, or by hematogenous spread from a distant site of infection. Infections of the paranasal sinuses, middle ear, and mastoid are the most common local events leading to brain abscess formation.[37–40] Brain abscesses arising secondary to paranasal sinus infection tend to occur in the frontal or temporal lobes by retrograde thrombophlebitis of the diploic veins. Osteomyelitic involvement of the frontal sinuses can extend directly into anterior and basal frontal lobes, whereas middle ear infections can extend directly by the transpetrous or translabyrinthine route to produce temporal lobe abscesses. Mastoid infections can extend directly into the temporal lobe or cerebellum or produce abscesses by retrograde thrombophlebitis of the emissary veins within the temporal bone.[41]

Unlike abscesses arising from direct extension, which tend to be solitary, metastatic brain abscesses arise from the hematogenous spread of microorganisms from a distant site of infection and tend to be multiple. These sites most often include infections of the skin, lungs, bone, oral cavity, and heart valves. Although abscesses of sinusitic or otitic origin tend to be superficial, metastatic abscesses tend to occur at the corticomedullary junction. Their distribution follows that of cerebral blood flow, thus regions of the frontal and parietal lobes supplied by the middle cerebral artery are most frequently involved. Less commonly, these abscesses are found in the thalamus, brainstem, and cerebellum. Interestingly, transient bacteremia does not appear to cause the brain abscesses; this probably results from the blood–brain barrier's resistance to infection.

Congenital heart disease in which cardiac malformations result in right-to-left shunting is another condition that predisposes to brain abscess formation.[42] Bypassing the pulmonary capillary bed where filtration normally occurs, bacteria may seed the brain and cause abscesses. This is exacerbated by the associated hypoxemia, polycythemia, and increased blood viscosity, which may lead to brain microinfarction and establish conditions conducive to bacterial growth and abscess formation.

Penetrating head trauma is another main cause of brain abscess.[43,44] Abscesses tend to develop soon after the trauma, although they may occur years later. Inoculation of the brain usually occurs from retained contaminated bone fragments and debris; bullets, heat-sterilized during their firing, tend not to cause brain contamination. Other avenues of post-traumatic infection include basilar skull fracture; subsequent CSF leak and meningitis may lead to brain inoculation with microorganisms. Prior craniotomy may result in the formation of brain abscesses when microorganisms may be inadvertently introduced during surgery or by direct spread from wound or osteomyelitic infections of the cranial bone flap. In these cases, the infected bone flap must be removed to cure the infection.

Finally, immune system compromise, from either chronic steroid or other immunosuppressive drug administration, the administration of cytotoxic chemotherapeutic agents, or HIV infection, can predispose to the development of brain abscesses from opportunistic processes. The opportunistic infections tend to be fungal, protozoal or viral, and arise from the reactivation of latent infection rather than de novo infection with these pathogens.[45]

The microbiology of brain abscesses has changed considerably during the past several decades. Although the incidence of streptococcal abscesses has remained about the same, there has been a significant decrease in the number caused by *Staphylococcus aureus*.[38,46] Gram-negative infection, however, has been increasing in incidence, as have those caused by anaerobic bacteria. Of the aerobic bacteria causing brain abscesses, staphylococcal, streptococcal, enterobacterial, and *Haemophilus* species predominate. Mixed infections may occur in up to one-third of cases.

The causative microorganisms of brain abscesses tends to be related to the initial site of infection. Thus, otitic and dental infections tend to cause anaerobic bacterial abscesses.[47,48] Sinusitic infections tend to give rise to *Staphylococcus aureus*, aerobic streptococcal, and *Haemophilus influenzae* abscesses; more than half are co-infected with anaerobic bacteria.[49] Metastatic abscesses tend to be caused by anaerobic bacteria. Pulmonary infections can give rise to a multiplicity of offending organisms, whereas cardiac infection often gives rise to streptococcal brain abscesses. In patients with AIDS or other immunocompromised states, fungal abscesses (*Cryptococcus neoformans*) and parasitic abscesses (*Toxoplasma gondii*) predominate.[50]

DIAGNOSIS

About 80 percent of patients with brain abscesses have a known clinical factor predisposing to the development of the abscess.[40,51,52] Other specific clinical features are not common. Although brain abscesses occur as a result of infection, only about 50 percent present with fever, usually of a low grade. Fevers of greater than 38.5°C suggest concomitant meningitis or systemic infection.[51] The symptoms related to brain abscesses depend largely on their size and location, and are often indistinguishable from those caused by other space-occupying lesions. Symptoms related to elevated intracranial pressure are common. Thus, headache is a significant feature in more than 70 percent of cases, and nausea and vomiting occur in 25 percent to 50 percent of cases.[39,40,53,54] Alterations of consciousness occur in two-thirds of patients with brain abscesses. Focal neurological deficits, the nature of which is related to the location of the infection, occur in 60 percent of cases. These include hemiparesis, dysphasia, visual field defects, ataxia, and nystagmus. Seizures occur in 30 percent to 50 percent of patients.[37,39,40,55] The timing of symptoms and their progression may help to differentiate brain abscesses from other intracranial processes, such as tumors.[56] Thus, symptoms related to brain abscesses tend to be of rapid onset and progression; they are usually present less than 2 weeks before medical evaluation. In the immunocompromised patient, however, symptoms may be of insidious onset and slowly progressive.

In general, laboratory tests are of little value in the diagnosis of brain abscesses. The peripheral white blood cell count is usually less than 15,000 cells/mm^3; only 30 percent of patients have white blood cell counts greater than 11,000 cell/mm^3. Less than 10 percent of patients have white blood cell counts greater than 20,000 cells/mm^3. This reflects the presence of concomitant systemic infection or meningitis.[39,51,57] In 90 percent of patients, the erythrocyte sedimentation rate is elevated to an average of about 50 mm/h. CSF examination is equally unhelpful in making the diagnosis of brain abscess. Reflecting elevated intracranial pressure, the opening pressure is often elevated. Unless complicated by meningitis, brain abscesses are associated with only a mild CSF pleocytosis, with a white blood cell count of less than 100 cells/mm³. CSF protein concentration is usually only mildly elevated (<100 mg/dl) and glucose concentration is often normal. Cultures of the CSF are usually negative. In the light of the nonspecific findings of CSF evaluation and the danger of herniation from elevated intracranial pressure, lumbar puncture should generally be avoided in these patients.

The CT radiologic appearance of the brain abscesses correlates with the stages of abscess development.[58,59] During the period of cerebritis, CT scans reveal an area of low density consistent with necrosis; patterns of contrast enhancement are inconsistent. During the capsule stage, noncontrast CT scans reveal a subtle ring around the region of low density consistent with the developing capsule. After contrast administration, this capsule enhances and tends to be thinnest along its medial border. T_1-weighted MRIs reveal a central region of marked low intensity surrounded by a discrete ring, which is isointense to mildly hyperintense. This is surrounded by a region of mild hypointensity. These regions correlate with the necrotic center, the abscess capsule, and surrounding brain edema. T_2-weighted MRIs reveal a central region of iso- to hyperintensity and a discrete ring of hypointensity surrounded by a zone of hyperintensity.[60-62]

Several different intracranial processes are included in the differential diagnosis of brain abscesses, including malignant brain tumors and infarcts. The diagnosis of brain abscess is suggested but not confirmed by the presence of an asymmetric capsule, multiple lesions, the location of the lesion(s) at the corticomedullary junction, and associated leptomeningeal enhancement.[41] Radionuclide imaging with ^{111}In-labeled white blood cells can help to distinguish brain abscesses from other intracranial space-occupying lesions.[63,64] Ultimately, aspiration/biopsy is often necessary to confirm the diagnosis of brain abscess.

MANAGEMENT

As with all infectious diseases, the choice of antibiotic therapy for the treatment of brain abscesses should be based on the results of culture and sensitivity testing. Of particular importance to the treatment of brain abscesses, however, is the ability of a given antibiotic to penetrate brain tissue. Most of the information available on the antibiotic penetration into the CNS comes from evaluation of CSF; antibiotic concentrations in the CSF and brain tissue do not always correlate well.[45,48,65-67] Antibiotics that have been shown to enter the brain at high concentration include chloramphenicol, selected third-generation cephalosporins, metronidazole, methicillin, nafcillin, penicillin, thimethoprim/ sulfamethoxasole, and vancomycin. Despite bacteriocidal concentrations of these antibiotics, bacteria may still be cultured from abscess aspirates, probably because of the acidic environment favoring bacterial growth and inhibiting antibiotic action.[65]

When direct culture results are pending or when they are impossible to obtain, empiric antibiotic therapy is based on the presumed pathogenesis of the brain abscess. Thus, abscesses of sinusitic origin frequently contain streptococcus and obligate anaerobes; agents effective against these bacteria should be chosen. Abscesses of otitic origin often contain mixed aerobic and anaerobic bacteria, while metastatic abscesses can involve a wide variety of organisms; thus, multiple broad-spectrum antibiotics are needed for empiric therapy. Post-traumatic brain abscesses usually involve *Staphylococcus aureus*, requiring therapy with vancomycin or a semisynthetic penicillinase-resistant penicillin.

The use of corticosteroids in the setting of brain abscesses remains somewhat controversial. Corticosteroids are effective at decreasing mass effect from associated cerebral edema, but at the same time significantly inhibit several factors involved with the host response to infection. They decrease fibroblast and leukocyte migration, limiting the effective response to infection and delaying abscess capsule formation.[68,69] Furthermore, they decrease contrast enhancement of the abscess capsule on CT scans, making it difficult to determine the response to antiobiotic therapy.[58] It has therefore been recommended that corticosteroids not be used in the setting of brain abscess unless patients are at risk of herniation or progressive neurological deficit from large masses..

In his first descriptions of brain abscesses, Macewen[70] proposed surgical therapy. In 1926, Dandy[71] first reported aspiration of a brain abscess through a burr hole, and in 1936, Vincent[72] reported successful excision of a brain abscess. From that time until recently, surgery has been the preferred method of managing brain abscesses. In the 1970s, however, several groups reported successful nonsurgical therapy of brain abscesses with antibiotics alone.[52,73–79] These investigators showed that the results of empiric antibiotic therapy were equal to those of surgery, with an overall success rate of 74 percent and mortality of 4 percent.[79]

This approach relies on the close clinical and radiologic follow-up of patients. Antibiotics are given for 6 weeks; during therapy, radiologic studies are performed on a weekly basis. At the completion of therapy, images are obtained monthly until all areas of abnormal enhancement resolve. The changes on radiographic study tend to lag behind clinical changes; generally, abscesses decrease in size after 2 to 3 weeks of therapy, and complete resolution usually takes 3 to 4 months, although it may take as long as 1 year.[56,80] Residual enhancement on radiologic studies is usually a sign of permanent cerebral injury and is of little pathologic significance, although it may rarely be a predictor of recurrence.

A critical review of the nonsurgical studies, however, reveals important differences between those patients treated surgically and those treated with antibiotics alone. Those treated "medically" had smaller abscesses and more frequently had deep-seated abscesses that would not be amenable to surgical therapy. The data suggest that large abscesses (>2.5 cm) are not cured by antibiotics alone.[65,78] Other problems may arise from this approach as well. The combined use of several antibiotics in the long term, as is frequently done in these cases, may allow for the uncontrolled growth of resistant organisms or may lead to greater toxicity to the patient. Depending on the microbiology of the abscess, such combination antibiotic therapy might not be necessary. Furthermore, the clinical and radiologic diagnosis of brain abscess is not always certain, and cases of mistaken antibiotic therapy of brain tumors have occurred.

With the advent of image-guided stereotactic techniques, aspiration of brain abscesses can be performed quickly and safely.[41,57,80–82] The procedure can be performed under local anesthesia and is of little trauma to the surrounding brain. Aspiration provides for diagnostic material and immediate decompression, with resultant decrease in intracranial pressure; by removing acidic and hypoxic necrotic material, it provides a more favorable environment for antibiotic therapy.[65,81]

Open surgical drainage or abscess excision remains a viable therapeutic option.[40,83] Although aspiration is preferable for lesions in the cerebritis stages, multiple lesions, deep-seated lesions, or lesions in eloquent regions, in some cases open surgical therapy remains attractive. Fungal abscesses tend to be cured only by surgical excision, but multiloculated abscesses may be incompletely drained by aspiration and require excision.[36] Post-traumatic abscesses often contain contaminated foreign bodies that, if retained, can lead to recurrence.[43,44]

RESULTS OF THERAPY

Although the classic literature reports an overall mortality of 50 percent, there has been a significant reduction in mortality with advances in the diagnosis and treatment of brain abscesses. At the University of California, San Francisco, for example, the mortality rate was 41 percent between 1970 and 1974; it fell to 9 percent between 1975 and 1980.[57] Improvement in microbiologic isolation techniques, more effective antibiotics, and the advent of neuroimaging techniques, such as CT and MRI, have resulted in earlier diagnosis and more effective treatment at stages when patients are, neurologically, relatively well.

The most significant predictor of response to therapy is the neurological condition of the patient on presentation.[39,40,51,54,57] Those who are awake and alert tend to do well, while patients who present stuporous or in a coma have a high mortality. Patients with slowly progressive symptoms tend to do better than those with a rapidly deteriorating course.[84] Abscesses of sinusitic or otitic origin tend to respond better than those of metastatic origin, presumably to their frequent multiplicity and involvement of deep brain structure.[36,37,39,84,85] When patients die during therapy, it is usually due to herniation from untreated mass effect or from abscess rupture into the ventricular system.[36,37]

Recurrence of brain abscesses occurs in 5 percent to 10 percent of patients, despite apparently adequate therapy.[36,40,51] Most abscesses recur within 6 weeks after therapy, although recurrence has been reported years later. Reasons for recurrence may include the use of inappropriate or insufficient antibiotics, the failure to aspirate or excise large abscesses, the presence of retained contaminated foreign bodies, and the failure to fully treat distant sites of infection.[41] The long-term morbidity associated with successful therapy includes seizures, cognitive dysfunction, and focal neurological deficits.[37,51] Seizures occur in 30 percent to 50 percent of patients; thus long-term prophylactic anticonvulsants may be indicated.[37,39,40,55] Fully half of patients may have permanent neurological deficits; 35 percent have hemiparesis related to the parietal location of many abscesses.

PROTOCOL FOR THE TREATMENT

The protocol developed by Osenbach and Loftus[85a] is quite sound and reflects the general consensus of the clinical neuroscience community. Most significantly, this protocol should be used as a general outline for therapy; each case must be considered separately, and care individualized to the needs of the patient.

When a brain abscess is suspected, urgent CT, MRI, or ultrasound guided aspiration is performed. In cases of multiple abscesses, the most safely accessible abscess is aspirated. Preoperative antibiotics, which increase the risk of sterile cultures, are not given. Antibiotic therapy as directed by culture and sensitivity data is given for 6 weeks. Neuroimaging studies are obtained at weekly intervals during therapy and monthly thereafter until the abscess has resolved. Open excision of abscesses is limited to large lesions at risk of causing herniation, which are well encapsulated and in noneloquent regions.

HUMAN IMMUNODEFICIENCY VIRUS-ASSOCIATED NEUROLOGICAL DISORDERS

The spectrum of neurological disease that complicates HIV-1 is diverse. Any part of the neuraxis may be affected. These illnesses can be classified into those that result from a direct involvement of the nervous system by HIV-1 and those that result from the associated immunologic abnormalities. In the latter category, infectious complications are the most common but not the sole cause of neurological disability. Other causes of neurological disease seen in association with the immunosuppression of HIV-1 infection include primary and metastatic neoplasms, metabolic-nutritional disorders, and cerebrovascular complications.

MENINGITIS

Acute HIV-1 meningitis[86,87] or meningoencephalitis[88] may accompany the acute viral illness following HIV-1 infection by 3 to 6 weeks. Systemic features of this acute illness include fever, generalized lymphadenopathy, pharyngeal injection, splenomegaly and splenic tenderness, maculopapular rash, and urticaria.[86,89] As serologic tests for antibodies to HIV-1 require 8 to 12 weeks to become positive, the ELISA and Western blot are negative. This meningitis is similar to other viral meningitides, characterized by headache, meningismus, photophobia, generalized seizures, and altered mental state. CSF examination reveals an increased protein (<100 mg %), a mononuclear pleocytosis (≤200 cells/mm^3) and normal glucose.[87] HIV-1 can be isolated from the CSF. In a small percentage of affected individuals, symptoms persist for months, but typically they are self-limited.

Other forms of infectious meningitis are observed with HIV-1 infection. In general, these meningitides occur in association with significant immunosuppression and are considered AIDS-defining illnesses. The most common are due to *Cryptococcus neoformans* and *Mycobacteria tuberculosis*. Despite severe cellular immunosuppression, meningitis due to *Listeria monocytogenes* is not observed as frequently as with equal degrees of immunosuppression accompanying lymphoproliperative states and other malignancies. Syphilitic meningitis and meningoencephalitis also occur with increased frequency in HIV-1 infection. The presence of concomitant skin rash and uveitis should suggest the diagnosis.[90]

MASS LESIONS

A decline in level of consciousness generally occurs in association with focal neurological abnormalities in the setting of HIV-1 infection as a result of a mass lesion of the brain, usually opportunistic infections or lymphoma. Occasionally, cerebral infarction due to HIV-1-related causes also may present as a mass lesion. The altered level of consciousness observed is typically the result of incipient brain herniation, which requires prompt intervention (as described for other causes of brain herniation).

Alternatively, mass lesions result in focal neurological disturbances, such as hemianopsia, hemiparesis, and hemianesthesia, in the absence of an alteration of level of consciousness. The most common opportunistic infection resulting in a mass lesion is toxoplasmosis, and the most common neoplasm is primary CNS lymphoma. In the presence of a suspected mass lesion, either a cranial MRI with gadolinium or a double-dose delayed brain CT is required. The former is more sensitive, but brain CT scan is more specific, particularly with respect to toxoplasmosis.[91] These studies often prove to be complementary.

Toxoplasmosis is the most common cause of intracerebral mass lesion occurring in association with HIV infection.[92,93] Toxoplasma encephalopathy may account for up to 40 percent of all neurological disease, depending on the geographic site of the study. In HIV-infected individuals with IgG toxoplasma antibody,[94] the risk of developing toxoplasmosis has been estimated at 6 percent to 12 percent. Fever and malaise preceding the onset of focal neurological deficits by several days to weeks are typical.[95] The most common focal finding is mild hemiparesis; headache and seizures are not unusual. Because of the predilection of the lesions for the basal ganglia, chorea may be observed, and has been said to be virtually pathognomonic of toxoplasmosis.[96] The course of the illness is typically subacute, with symptoms arising over the course of 1 to 2 weeks.

Brain CT typically reveals multiple nodular or ring-enhancing lesions with edema and mass effect and a predilection for the basal ganglia and frontoparietal lobes.[95,97,98] However, the lesions may be nonenhancing dense on occasion. The most helpful study in identifying lesions for biopsy or following the progression of the disease is double-dose delayed CT scan with axial thin sections. Although less sensitive than MRI, the CT scan is superior in gauging the activity of lesions and in distinguishing lesions in close proximity to one another. CSF findings in these patients are nonspecific, and brain biopsy is the only unequivocal means to establish the diagnosis. A trial of antitoxoplasmosis therapy of 2 weeks duration in those patients with suspected toxoplasma encephalitis is warranted before resorting to brain biopsy. The therapy of toxoplasma encephalitis is oral pyrimethamine (an initial loading dose of 50 to 100 mg, followed by 25 mg/day) and 6 to 8 g sulfadiazine per day divided into four equal doses. These patients are monitored clinically and by radiographic criteria for resolution of their lesions. When the antitoxoplasmosis regimen fails to effect clinical and radiographic improvement, brain biopsy should be performed. Corticosteroids administration should be avoided, if possible, as it may confuse the interpretation of this therapeutic trial.

REFERENCES

1. Davey PG, Cruickshank JK, McManus IC et al: Bacterial meningitis—ten years experience. J Hygiene 88:383, 1982
2. Schlech WF, Ward JI, Band JD et al: Bacterial meningitis in the United States. 1978 through 1981. The National Bacterial Meningitis Surveillance Study. JAMA 253:1749, 1985
3. Smith AL: Neurologic sequelae of meningitis. N Engl J Med 319:1012, 1988
4. Barson WJ, Miller MA, Brady MY, Powell DA: Prospective comparative trial of ceftriaxone vs. conventional therapy for treatment of bacterial meningitis in children. Pediatr Infect Dis 4:362, 1985
5. Cherubin CE, Marr JS, Sierra MF, Becker S: *Listeria* and gram negative bacillary meningitis in New York City, 1972–1979. Frequent causes of meningitis in adults. Am J Med 71:199, 1981
6. Cadoz M, Denis F, Liop Mar J: Étude epidemiologique des cas de meningitis purulentes hospitalises á Dakar pendant la decennie 1970–1979. Bull WHO 59:575, 1981
7. Feldman WE: Relation of concentrations of bacteria and bacterial antigen in cerebrospinal fluid to prognosis in patients with bacterial meningitis. N Engl J Med 296:433, 1977
8. Del Rio M, Chrane D, Shelton D et al: Ceftriaxone vs. ampicillin and chloramphenicol for treatment of bacterial meningitis in children. Lancet i:1241, 1983
9. Editorial: Steroids and meningitis. Lancet ii:1307, 1989
10. Tunkel AR, Wispelwey B, Scheld WM: Bacterial meningitis: recent advances in pathophysiology and treatment. Ann Intern Med 112:610, 1990

11. Greenwood BM: Chemotactic activity of cerebrospinal fluid in pyogenic meningitis. J Clin Pathol 31:213, 1978
12. Wyler DJ, Wasserman SI, Karchmer AW: Substances which modulate leukocyte migration are present in CSF during meningitis. Ann Neurol 5:322, 1979
13. Schleimer RP, Rutledge BK: Cultured human vascular endothelial cells acquire adhesiveness for neutrophils after stimulation with interleukin 1, endotoxin and tumor-promoting phorbol diesters. J Immunol 136:649, 1986
14. Thomas PD, Hampson FW, Casale JM, Hunninghake GW: Neutrophil adherence to human endothelial cells. J Lab Clin Med 111:286, 1988
15. Bevilacqua MP, Pober JS, Wheller ME et al: Interleukin 1 acts on cultured human vacular endothelium to increase the adhesion of polymorphonuclear leukocytes, monocytes, and related leukocyte cell lines. J Clin Invest 76:2003, 1985
16. Varani J, Bendelow J, Sealey DE et al: Tumor necrosis factor enhances susceptibility of vascular endothelial cells to neutrophil-mediated killing. Lab Invest 59:292, 1988
17. Mustafa MM, Ramilo O, Olsen DK et al: Tumor necrosis factor in mediating experimental *Haemophilus influenzae* type b meningitis. J Clin Invest 84: 1253, 1989
18. Libby P, Ordovas JM, Auger KR et al: Endotoxin and tumor necrosis factor induce interleuken-1 gene expression in adult human vascular endothelial cells. Am J Pathol 124:179, 1986
19. Miossec P, Cavender D, Ziff M: Production of interleukin 1 by human endothelial cells. J Immunol 136:2486, 1986
20. Editorial: *Cryptococcus* in AIDS. Lancet 25:1434, 1988
21. Waage A, Halstensen A, Espevik T: Association between tumour necrosis factor in serum and fatal outcome in patients with meningococcal disease. Lancet i:355, 1987
22. Davis LE: Acute bacterial meningitis. p. 135. In Wiener W (ed): Emergent and Urgent Neurology. JB Lippincott, Philadelphia, 1992
23. Taylor HG, Michaels RH, Mazur PM et al: Intellectual, neuropsychological, and achievement outcomes in children six to eight years after recovery from *Haemophilus influenzae* meningitis. Pediatrics 74:198, 1984
24. Adams RD, Victor M: Nonviral infections of the nervous system. p. 554. In: Principles of Neurology. 4th Ed. McGraw Hill, New York, 1989
25. Kales CP, Holzman RS: Listeriosis in patients with HIV infection: clinical manifestations and response to therapy. J AIDS 3:139, 1990
26. DeJong RN: Miscellaneous neurologic signs. p. 482. In: The Neurologic Examination. 4th Ed. Harper & Row, Hagerstown, MD, 1979
27. Fishman RA: Cerebrospinal Fluid in Diseases of the Nervous System. WB Saunders, Philadelphia, 1980
28. Scheld WM: Bacterial meningitis in the patient at risk: intrinsic factors and host defense mechanisms. Am J Med (suppl. 1):193, 1984
29. Quagliarello VJ, Scheld WM: Bacterial infections in adults. p. 1384. In Asbury AK, McKhann GM, McDonald, WI (eds): Diseases of the Nervous System. Vol. 2. WB Saunders, Philadelphia, 1986
30. Kaplan SL, Feigin RD: The syndrome of inappropriate antidiuretic hormone in children with bacterial meningitis. J Pediatr 92:758, 1978
31. Roos KL: Dexamethasone and nonsteroidal anti-inflammatory agents in the treatment of bacterial meningitis. Clin Ther 12:290, 1990
32. Escobar JA, Belsey MA, Duenas A et al: Mortality from tuberculosis meningitis reduced by steroid therapy. Pediatrics 56:1050, 1975

33. O'Toole RD, Thornton GF, Mukherjee MK, Nath RL: Dexamethasone in tuberculosis meningitis. Relationship of cerebrospinal fluid effects to therapeutic efficacy. Ann Intern Med 70:39, 1969

34. Lebel MH, Freij BJ, Syrogiannopoulos GA et al: Dexamethasone therapy for bacterial meningitis. N Engl J Med 319:964, 1988

35. Odio CM, Faingezicht I, Paris M et al: The beneficial effects of early dexamethasone administration in infants and children with bacterial meningitis. N Engl J Med 324:1525, 1991

36. Britt RH: Brain abscess. p. 1928. In Wilkins RH, Rengarchary SS (eds): Neurosurgery. McGraw-Hill, New York, 1985

37. Beller AJ, Sahar A, Praiss I: Brain abscess. Review of 89 cases over a period of 30 years. J Neurol Psychiatry 36:757, 1973

38. Garfield J: Management of supratentorial intracranial abscess: a review of 200 cases. 2:7, 1969

39. Morgan H, Wood MW, Murphy F: Experiments with 88 consecutive cases of brain abscess. J Neurosurg 38:698, 1973

40. Samson DS, Clark K: A current review of brain abscess. Am J Med 54:201, 1973

41. Osenbach R, Loftus C: Diagnosis and management of brain abscess. p. 403. In Haines S, Hall W (eds): Neurosurgery Clinics of North America: Infections of Neurological Surgery. Vol. 3. WB Saunders, Philadelphia, 1992

42. Fisher EG, McLennan JE, Suzuki Y: Cerebral abscess in children. Am J Dis Child 135:746, 1981

43. Hagan RE: Early complications following penetrating wounds of the brain. J Neurosurg 34:132, 1971

44. Rish BL, Caveness WF, Dillon JD et al: Analysis of brain abscess after pentrating craniocerebral injuries in Vietnam. Neurosurgery 9:535, 1981

45. Levy RM, Gutin PH, Baskin DS et al: Vancomycin penetration of a brain abscess: case report and review of the literature. Neurosurgery 18:632, 1986

46. Nielsen H, Harmsen A, Gyldensted C: Cerebral abscess. A long-term follow-up. Acta Neurol Scand 67:330, 1983

47. Alderson D, Strong AJ, Ingham HR et al: Fifteen-year review of the mortality of brain abscess. Neurosurgery 8:1, 1981

48. De Louvois J: The bacteriology and chemotherapy of brain abscess. J Antimicrob Chemother 4:395, 1978

49. Wispelwey B, Scheld WM: Brain abscess. p. 777. In Mandell GL, Douglas RG Jr, Bennett JE (eds): Principles and Practice of Infectious Diseases. 3rd Ed. Churchill Livingstone, New York, 1990

50. Levy RM, Bredesen DE, Rosenblum ML: Neurological manifestations of the acquired immunodeficiency syndrome (AIDS): experience at UCSF and review of the literature. J Neurosurg 62:475, 1985

51. Carey ME, Chou SN, French LA: Experience with brain abscesses. J Neurosurg 36:1, 1972

52. Rosenblum JL, Hoff JT, Norman D et al: Decreased mortality from brain abscess since advent of computerized tomography. J Neurosurg 49:658, 1978

53. Nielsen H, Carsten G, Harmsen A: Cerebral abscess. Aetiology and pathogenesis, symptoms, diagnosis and treatment. A review of 200 cases from 1935–1976. Acta Neurol Scand 65:609, 1982

54. Yang SY: Brain abscess: a review of 400 cases. J Neurosurg 55:794, 1981

55. Carey ME, Chou SN, French LA: Long-term neurological residua in patients surviving brain abscess with surgery. J Neurosurg 34:652, 1971

56. Whelan MA, Hilal SK: Computed tomography as a guide in the diagnosis and follow-up of brain abscesses. Radiology 135:663, 1980
57. Mamapalam TH, Rosenblum ML: Trends in the management of bacterial brain abscesses: a review of 102 cases over 17 years. Neurosurgery 23:451, 1988
58. Britt RH, Enzmann DR: Clinical stages of human brain abscesses on serial CT scans after contrast infusion. Computerized tomographic, neuropathological and clinical correlations. J Neurosurg 59:972, 1983
59. Enzmann DR, Britt RH, Placone R: Staging of human brain abscess by computed tomography. Radiology 146:703, 1983
60. Brant-Zawadzki M, Enzmann DR, Placone RC et al: NMR imaging of experimental brain abscess: comparison with CT. AJNR 4:250, 1983
61. Haimes AB, Zimmerman RD, Morgello S et al: MR imaging of brain abscesses. AJNR 10:270, 1989
62. Sze G, Zimmerman RD: The magnetic resonance imaging of infections and inflammatory diseases. Radiol Clin North Am 26:839, 1988
63. Rehncrona S, Brismar J, Holtas S: Diagnosis of brain abscess with indium-111-labelled leukocytes. Neurosurgery 16:23, 1985
64. Bellotti C, Arango MG, Medina M et al: Differential diagnosis of CT-hypodense cranial lesions with indium 111-oxine-labeled leukocytes. J Neurosurg 64:750, 1986
65. Black P, Graybill JR, Charache P: Penetration of brain abscess by systemically administered antibiotics. J Neurosurg 38:706, 1973
66. De Louvois J, Gortvai P, Hurley R: Bacteriology of abscesses of the central nervous system: a multicentre prospective study. Br Med J [Clin Res] 2:981, 1977
67. Everett ED, Strausbaugh LJ: Antimicrobial agents and the central nervous system. Neurosurgery 6:691, 1980
68. Quartey GRC, Johnston JA, Rozdilsky B: Decadron in the treatment of cerebral abscess: an experimental study. J Neurosurg 45:301, 1976
69. Bohl I, Wallenfang T, Bothe H et al: The effect of glucocorticoids in the combined treatment experimental brain abscess in cats. Adv Neurosurg 9:125, 1981
70. Macewen W: Pyrogenic Infective Diseases of the Brain and Spinal Cord. J Maclehose and Sons, Glasgow, 1983
71. Dandy WE: Treatment of chronic abscess of the brain by tapping: preliminary note. JAMA 87:1477, 1926
72. Vincent C: Sur une methode de traitment des abces subaigus des hemispheres cerebraux: large desompression, puis ablation enmasse sans drainage. Gaz Med Fr 43:93, 1936
73. Heineman HS, Braude AI: Intracranial suppurative disease. JAMA 218:1542, 1971
74. Barsoum AH, Lewis HC, Cannillo KL: Nonoperative treatment of multiple brain abscesses. Surg Neurol 16:283, 1981
75. Berg B, Franklin G, Cunoe R et al: Non-surgical cure of brain abscess: early diagnosis and follow-up with computerized tomography. Ann Neurol 3:474, 1978
76. Bloom WH, Tuazon CU: Successful treatment of multiple brain abscesses with antibiotics alone. Rev Infect Dis 7:189, 1985
77. Burke LP, Ho SU, Cerullo LJ et al: Multiple brain abscesses. Surg Neurol 16:452, 1981
78. Rosenblum JL, Hoff JT, Norman D et al: Non-operative treatment of brain abscesses in selected high-risk patients. J Neurosurg 52:217, 1980
79. Rosenblum ML, Mampalam TJ, Pons VG: Controversies in the management of brain abscesses. Clin Neurosurg 33:603, 1986

80. Dobkin JF, Healton EB, Dickinson T et al: Nonspecificity of ring enhancement in "medically cured" brain abscesses. Neurology 34:139, 1984

81. Dyste GN, Hitchon RW, Menezes AH et al: Stereotaxic surgery in the treatment of multiple brain abscesses. J Neurosurg 69:188, 1988

82. Miller ES, Dias PS, Uttley D: CT scanning in the management of intracranial abscess: a review of 100 cases. 2:439, 1988

83. Taylor J: The case for excision in the treatment of brain abscess. Br J Neurosurg 1:173, 1987

84. Brewer NS, MacCarty CS, Wellman WE: Brain abscess: a review of recent experience. Ann Intern Med 82:571, 1975

85. Wood M, Anderson M: Suppuration and focal disease. p. 249. In Wood M, Anderson M (eds): Neurological Infections. WB Saunders, Philadelphia, 1988

85a. Osenbach RK, Loftus CM: Diagnosis and management of brain abscess. Neurosurg Clin N Amer 3:403, 1992

86. Bessen LJ, Greene JB, Louie E: Severe polynyositis-like syndrome associated with zidovudine therapy of AIDS and ARC. (letter) N Engl J Med 318:708, 1988

87. Bishopric G, Bruner J, Butler J: Guillain-Barre syndrome with cytomegalovirus infection of peripheral nerve. Arch Pathol Lab Med 109:1106, 1985

88. Bredesen DE, Messing R: Neurological syndrome heralding the acquired immunodeficiency syndrome (abstract). Ann Neurol 14:141, 1983

89. Bishburg E, Sunderm G, Reichman LB et al: Central nervous system tuberculosis with the acquired immunodeficiency syndrome and its related complex. Ann Intern Med 105:210, 1986

90. Katz D, Berger JR: Neurosyphillis in AIDS. Arch Neurol 46:895, 1989

91. Post MJD, Berger JR, Hensley GT: The radiology of central nervous system disease in acquired immunodeficiency syndrome. p. 1. In Taveras JM, Ferrucci KT (eds): Radiology: Diagnosis-Imaging-Intervention, JB Lippincott, Philadelphia, 1988

92. Maier H, Budka H, Lassman H et al: Vacuolar myelopathy with multinucleated giant cells in the acquired immunodeficiency virus (HIV) antigens. Acta Neuropathol 78:497, 1989

93. Whiteman M, Post MJD, Berger JR et al: PML in 45 HIV + Patients: Neuroimaging with Pathologic Correlation. Presented at the 77th Scientific Assembly and Annual Meeting of the RSNA, Dec 1–6, 1991

94. Wong B, Gold JWM, Brown AE et al: Central nervous system toxoplasmosis in homosexual men parenteral drug abusers. Ann Intern Med 100:36, 1984

95. Navia BA, Jordan BD, Price RW: The AIDS dementia complex: I. Clinical features. Ann Neurol 19:517, 1986

96. Nath A, Jankovic J, Pettigrew LC: Movement disorders and AIDS. Neurology 37:37, 1987

97. Leport C, Vilde JL, Katlama C et al: Toxoplasmose cerebrale de l'immunodeprime: diagnostic et traitement. Ann Med Interne 138:30, 1987

98. Post MJD, Chan JC, Hensley GT et al: Toxoplasma encephalitis in Haitian adults with acquired immunodeficiency syndrome: a clinical-pathologic-CT correlation. AJNR 4:155, 1983

99. Sanford JP: Guide to Antimicrobial Therapy 1992. University of Texas Southwestern Medical School, Division of Infectious Diseases, Department of Internal Medicine. Antimicrobial Therapy Inc., Dallas, TX, 1992

10

Difficult Behaviors

Jeffrey L. Clothier
Hilton R. Lacy

The management of critically ill patients is often complicated by the behavioral responses of the patient. Difficult to manage behaviors may indicate either pre-existing psychiatric illness, neuropsychiatric sequelae of the primary illness or its treatment, or the behavioral response of the patient to the treatment condition. None of these etiologies are mutually exclusive. Difficult to manage behaviors require a flexible and comprehensive approach. In many medical centers, psychiatric consultation facilitates the management of the difficult behaviors. It is the goal of this chapter to derive a model of behavior and an approach to managing these difficult behaviors. To do so, we review (1) the behavioral assessment of intensive care unit (ICU) patients, (2) behavioral responses to the ICU setting, and (3) pharmacologic and behavioral management techniques for specific types of problem behaviors.

The discussion of difficult behaviors is facilitated by psychiatric nomenclature. Several psychiatric conditions are seen in ICU patients. Organic and related mental conditions comprise approximately one-half of all ICU behavioral disorders.[1,2] The interaction of the psychiatric condition with the medical illness and treatment in the ICU complicates the evaluation process. Behavioral difficulties represent a breakdown in the patients' ability to maneuver efficiently in their environment. The behavior becomes problematic when it interferes with the ICU management. The manifestations of the problem behaviors range from personality clashes with staff to psychosis and delirium. The exact incidence of psychiatric problems in the ICU is not known. It is estimated that 30 percent to 60 percent of medically hospitalized patients will exhibit psychological dysfunction.[3] It may be more unusual to find a patient in the ICU who is free of behavioral difficulties.

Specific etiologies for behavioral disorders in the ICU are vast.[2,4,5] The specific behavior may be the result of the interaction of a sick body on a healthy mind (somatopsychic), a sick mind on a healthy body (psychosomatic), or a sick body on a sick mind (compound or complicated psychopathology). The symptoms produced are further influenced by the interaction of the patient

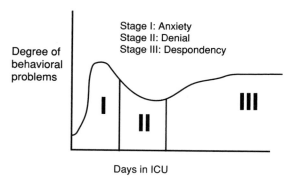

Fig. 10-1 Hypothetical response to ICU treatment in a patient.

with family, staff, other patients, and their environment. Also, ICUs character-istically care for specific populations, such as cardiac, cancer, and burn pa-tients. Such ICUs could expect different problem behaviors from units with less specific populations.[1,5] Clinicians should be cognizant of the effects of the medical conditions common to their unit and the effects of the technologies used in the unit on the neuropsychiatric functioning of their patients.

Admission to an ICU can have enduring psychological consequences. The response to an illness is magnified in the ICU setting. Figure 10-1 illustrates these phases. In general, the longer the stay in the ICU, the more enduring the behaviors. The initial phase of anxiety gives way to a period of denial, followed by despondency in many patients. It is the effect of the response in these states that is of importance in ICU patients. For instance, fear and anxiety associated with the initial days in a coronary care unit may represent an adverse effect on cardiac function because of the release of catecholamines. Organic mental disorders, such as delirium, can be associated with significant mortality during and after hospitalization.[2,6] Treatment of psychiatric comor-bid conditions is known to have beneficial effects on the length of stay and hospital costs. Despite the importance of effective management of these condi-tions, their detection is frequently overlooked.

ASSESSMENT OF THE DIMENSIONS OF BEHAVIOR

Problem behaviors may include regression to a point at which medical care is compromised. In beginning the approach to the behaviorally disordered patient, one must describe the behaviors in common terms. Behavior can be described along the dimensions of thought, affect, motility, intellect, and social activities. Functioning within these dimensions is normally congruent, in that specific perceptions and thoughts (e.g., seeing a snake) evoke specific emotions (e.g., fear) that are based on previously learned material (experi-ence). The end result is usually specific motoric behaviors (e.g., agitation) within the context of the environment. Acute organic illness may interfere with specific substrates of behaviors, such as memory and sensory processing, thus compromising the overall behavior of the patient. To assess functioning, the medical record should be reviewed and a standardized assessment of behavior performed.

Review of the medical record provides information regarding the known circumstances of admission and subsequent care. The first goal of treatment is to determine and correct the cause of the disordered behavior. A good medical record delineates behavior in specific terms. It is extremely useful for disorientation to be *described* rather than referred to simply as confusion. The documentation of behavior in the nurses' notes provides longitudinal information not available in a single interview. Careful description of behavior in the chart may disclose circadian alterations, which might suggest reduced arousal or "sundowning." The medical history may also provide clues regarding functioning prior to admission. Information regarding previous strokes, head injuries, etc., may suggest a compromised nervous system, which would be more susceptible to behavioral problems in the ICU. The medical record provides information regarding medications being used and medications to be avoided. The behavior in question can be evaluated against the starting and stopping of particular medications. The initial review of the record should also explain how the problem behavior is interfering with medical care, so that appropriate risk and benefits for interventions can be judged.

The social/developmental history may be particularly useful in predicting behavioral responses to stress and suggesting useful management strategies. Individuals develop a hierarchy of habit patterns and defenses against stress. A social/developmental history should survey areas of past stress and document the patient's behavioral responses. Periods that are typically stressful include graduation from school, marriage, divorce, loss of parents or spouse, military service, bankruptcy, and previous catastrophic illnesses. The patient's responses following such stresses should predict their response to the present stresses.

The formal mental status examination begins on meeting the patient. There are subjective and objective components. The subjective components are based on the examiner's cross-referencing observed behaviors in others. For instance, a patient's appearance, attitude, and affect are observable, but are described as appropriate or inappropriate based on the observer's criteria for normal appearance, attitude, and affect in patients in the ICU. The information gained in these observations may provide clues for more in-depth testing in other specific areas. Specific questions concerning the patient's attitude and emotional state should be attempted. Answers may be clarified as to the presence and extent of fear, sadness, anger, or euphoria. In discussing the patient's response to the ICU setting, specific questions concerning thoughts of self-harm, assaultive ideations, thoughts of special powers, or unusual sensations or experiences can be asked.

The objective component of the formal mental status examination requires evaluation of cognition and intellect. This will require formal assessment of the thought form, content, and learning/memory. The "mini-mental state examination"[7] (MMSE) is a widely used form of this part of the mental status examination. The MMSE is composed of a possible 30 points, testing orientation, memory, language, calculation, attention, and concentration, and constructional praxis (Table 10-1). A score of 24 or less is considered indicative of significant cognitive impairment. However, any incorrect responses may indicate possible organic impairment.[6] Although sensitive, the MMSE has limited specificity. However, the MMSE is a simple and rapid screening test that can contribute to the understanding of a behaviorally disordered patient. It should be given routinely to patients in ICU settings.

At the conclusion of the chart review and the formal mental status examination, the patient's behavior can be described on the five dimensions of behavior discussed above. Collateral information regarding the efficiency and integrity of central nervous system functioning should be sought. The bedside neuropsychiatric examination allows for a more comprehensive evaluation of the integrity of the nervous system than most screening neurological examinations. The core of the neuropsychiatric examination is the formal mental status examination and the screening neurological examination. The neuropsychiatric examination is extended to include a survey of higher cortical functioning. The details of a standard screening neurological examination are known to all physicians and are not discussed here. Instead, we focus on the bedside examination of the higher cortical functions.

The neurocortical examination divides the cortex into four principal lobes, as

---

Table 10-1. MINI-MENTAL STATE EXAMINATION

Orientation (day, date, month, season, year, state, county, city, hospital, floor)

Registration (three objects repeated back to examiner immediately)

Attention and concentration (serial 7's, count up to 5 or spell WORLD backward)

Recall short-term memory task (three objects given during registration task)

Language (name pencil and watch; repeat "no ifs, ands, or buts"; follow a three-step command; read and obey "close your eyes"; write a sentence)

Construction (copy a design: intersecting pentagons, observe angles)

Scoring
    Orientation task: 1 point for each element of orientation (maximum of 10 points)
    Registration task: 1 point for each item on first trial (maximum of 3 points)
    Attention and concentration task: 1 point for each correct subtraction or letter spelled (maximum of 5 points)
    Recall task: 1 point for each item remembered from the registration task (maximum of 3 points)
    Language tasks: (maximum for language tasks of 9 points)
        Naming pencil and watch: 1 point each (maximum of 2 points)
        Repetition: 1 point
        Three-step command: 1 point for each step (maximum of three points)
        Reading: 1 point
        Writing a sentence: 1 point if it is sensible and has a verb and subject
        Constructional praxis: 1 point if all 10 angles are present and two intersect

Total: maximum of 30 points; scores less than 24 are considered significant.

(From Folstein MF, et al.[7])

well as dominant and nondominant hemispheres. The specialized functioning common to these cortical regions can be described as language, motor, memory, and information processing functions. Figures 10-2 and 10-3 illustrate this division. The neurocortical examination provides a model for evaluating and following focal pathologies. Multifocal and diffuse pathologies can be differentiated from focal pathologies, which may aid in the differential diagnosis of acquired behavioral disorders.

The chart review, formal mental status examination, and neurocortical examination provide a framework to describe functioning in the five dimensions of behavior in longitudinal fashion, with reference to known or suspected insults to the substrate. The behavioral description can be thought of as a summary statement. For example, "A 25 year old married female status post motor vehicle accident 2 weeks ago with a previous history of depressive illness consulted for new onset of poor sleep, appetite, anhedonia, crying spells, reduced concentration and suicidal thoughts. The formal mental status examination and the neurocortical examination reveals dysphoria with a minimally reactive mood, mild expressive aphasia, asymmetric reflexes (R>L) and lateralized pathologic frontal reflexes, impaired concentration, attention and memory, with orientation to person and place only." Such a summary identifies the premorbid psychiatric history, evidence for a left anterior injury, and the depressive behaviors. This allows the clinician to consider a possible organic affective syndrome even in a patient with a history of depression.

The origins of the behavioral disturbance should be considered. The most crucial differential in dealing with patients with behavioral problems is whether the behavior is the result of a so-called organic brain syndrome or functional syndrome. It is important to recognize that such splitting suggests a mind–body dualism, which is artificial and may be counterproductive. It may be more beneficial to consider whether the behavior is acquired or developmental.

An acquired behavioral disorder is the result of insult to the organic substrate of the mind, and a developmental behavioral disorder is the result of the usual habit patterns or learned responses of the patient to stress. There are no pathognomonic signs to distinguish a developmental from an acquired behavioral disorder. In general, a patient with developmental behavioral disorders alone will exhibit stereotypic stress responses. That is to say that the patient's response to current stress is usually similar to the responses to prior stresses. Because these responses are based on a hierarchy, the sudden appearance of less well-organized defenses signals a loss of adaptation, and may suggest an acquired insult to the nervous system. For example, the literature is replete with reports of patients with a sudden onset of "conversion hysteria" in which organic etiologies are later discovered.[8] A common feature of such cases is usually the absence of previous conversion symptoms during adolescence and young adulthood (psychologically stressful times).

Following such a behavioral description, further testing can be performed to examine the hypothesis generated. The techniques available can be de-

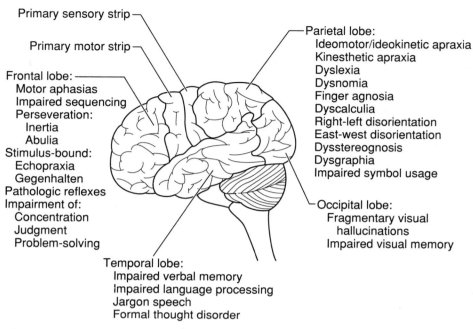

Primary sensory strip

Primary motor strip

Frontal lobe:
  Motor aphasias
  Impaired sequencing
  Perseveration:
    Inertia
    Abulia
  Stimulus-bound:
    Echopraxia
    Gegenhalten
  Pathologic reflexes
  Impairment of:
    Concentration
    Judgment
    Problem-solving

Parietal lobe:
  Ideomotor/ideokinetic apraxia
  Kinesthetic apraxia
  Dyslexia
  Dysnomia
  Finger agnosia
  Dyscalculia
  Right-left disorientation
  East-west disorientation
  Dysstereognosis
  Dysgraphia
  Impaired symbol usage

Occipital lobe:
  Fragmentary visual
    hallucinations
  Impaired visual memory

Temporal lobe:
  Impaired verbal memory
  Impaired language processing
  Jargon speech
  Formal thought disorder

Fig. 10-2 Dysfunctions caused by damage to left (dominant) hemisphere of brain.

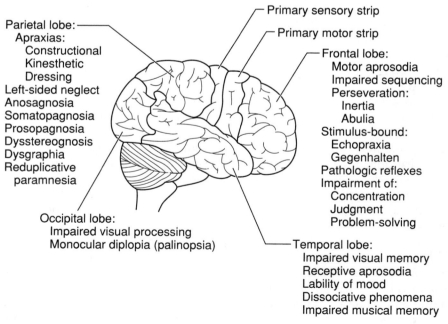

Primary sensory strip

Primary motor strip

Parietal lobe:
  Apraxias:
    Constructional
    Kinesthetic
    Dressing
  Left-sided neglect
  Anosagnosia
  Somatopagnosia
  Prosopagnosia
  Dysstereognosis
  Dysgraphia
  Reduplicative
    paramnesia

Frontal lobe:
  Motor aprosodia
  Impaired sequencing
  Perseveration:
    Inertia
    Abulia
  Stimulus-bound:
    Echopraxia
    Gegenhalten
  Pathologic reflexes
  Impairment of:
    Concentration
    Judgment
    Problem-solving

Occipital lobe:
  Impaired visual processing
  Monocular diplopia (palinopsia)

Temporal lobe:
  Impaired visual memory
  Receptive aprosodia
  Lability of mood
  Dissociative phenomena
  Impaired musical memory

Fig. 10-3 Dysfunctions caused by damage to right (nondominant) hemisphere of brain.

scribed as anatomic, physiologic, and psychological. Computed tomography and magnetic resonance imaging are the basic anatomic tests used to examine a behavioral hypotheses. However, these techniques provide mere anatomic and not physiologic data. Thus, disorders that affect neuronal metabolism may not be revealed by these techniques. Obviously, physiologic data are provided from peripheral and central nervous system laboratory data. Blood chemistry survey may disclose evidence of an extracranial cause of the behavior, such as hepatic or renal failure. Intracranial pathologies may be revealed by the use of more invasive laboratory techniques, such as lumbar puncture or cisternography. Noninvasive test for nonanatomic intracranial pathologies are limited to electroencephalography and possibly nuclear medicine evaluation of regional cerebral blood flow.

PROBLEM BEHAVIORS IN THE INTENSIVE CARE UNIT

As mentioned above, problem behaviors can range from personality clashes to frank psychosis and delirium in ICU patients. We consider here a hierarchy of severity. The severity is judged relative to the dangerousness of the behavior in the immediate term. Emergent behaviors commonly seen in the ICU setting include delirium, psychosis, depression with or without suicidality, and drug and alcohol withdrawal syndromes. Less emergent yet still problematic are the adjustment, anxiety, and characterologic disorders.

DELIRIUM ("ACUTE BRAIN FAILURE")

Delirium is the most common condition encountered by psychiatric consultants in the ICU setting.[1,9] It represents a rapid deterioration in the efficiency and integrity of functioning of the central nervous system. The hallmarks of delirium are usually the result of diffuse cerebral dysfunction. The most common etiologies of deliria are diffuse or multifocal and generally represent perfusion, metabolic, and toxic conditions.

Abrupt onset of confusion and clouding of consciousness with disruption of the normal processes of orientation and memory, arousal, attention, motility, affective regulation, perception, and cognition are the characteristic findings in delirious patients. The symptoms typically fluctuate throughout the day and are most pronounced in the evening and night. The disturbed arousal and disorientation of the patient, accompanied by agitation and auditory and visual hallucinations, typifies acute delirium of different etiologies. DSM-III R elaborates a list of diagnostic criteria for establishing the diagnosis.[10] The most important criteria are the clouding of consciousness and disturbed arousal. In their delirium, such patients may present a danger to themselves and others because of their misperception of the environment. Thus, therapeutic interventions require protection of the patients from themselves.

The model of the determinants of behavior described above allows the clinician to identify patients at particular risk of developing a delirium. Patients with previously compromised nervous system, such as demented patients, substance-abusing patients, and traumatic brain-injured patients, are at increased risk for developing a delirium in the ICU.[1–3,5] Such patients have limited adaptational reserves and decompensate quickly in the ICU setting.

Management of Delirium

The management of delirium requires prompt identification of the cause. Also, it requires protecting the patients from injuring themselves or others. In general, the management is divided into diagnostic, therapeutic, and environmental. Diagnostically emergent and urgent disorders should be considered. Delirium represents acute brain failure. Although several potential etiologies exist, the clinician should have a hierarchy for consideration of potentially fatal causes, such as infection, intoxications, rapidly expanding intracranial masses, electrolyte disturbances, and effects of other organ system failures, such as hypoxia and uremia. The mortality associated with delirium suggests an urgency to the evaluation. It is estimated that 40 percent to 50 percent of delirious patients will die within 1 year.[2] The evaluation therefore will require laboratory studies as well as a physical examination. Many of the causes of delirium may fluctuate during the course of a single day. Therefore, the laboratory diagnosis should be performed quickly.

Therapeutic interventions should be aimed first at stabilizing the behavior to minimize any adverse consequences of the behavior on the medical condition of the patient. Such interventions are basically two-pronged: pharmacologic and environmental. Unnecessary medications should be stopped. Several otherwise benign medications can have additive anticholinergic effects that worsen most deliria. Also, sedative-hypnotic agents should be avoided. These agents impair arousal and can paradoxically excite the delirious patient.[11] Most unmanageable behaviors can be treated with neuroleptic agents.[12] The calming effect of these agents is not the same as simple sedation. A general guideline can be to start low and go slow. However, in some situations rapid intervention is required to prevent deterioration in the ICU patient.[12]

As a group, neuroleptics can be divided into low-potency and high-potency. In general, low-potency neuroleptics are more sedating, but also have more effects on the cardiovascular system. However, high-potency neuroleptics have less sedation but few side effects on the cardiovascular system. In the majority of delirious patients in the ICU, the high-potency neuroleptics are chosen because of the lack of significant effects on the cardiovascular system. The most commonly used agent is haloperidol, although thiothixene can also be used.[6,12] Both agents also have the advantage of being available in parenteral forms. The typical dosing and side effects of haloperidol is shown in Figure 10-4. The primary goal is to titrate the favorable behavior against the side effects of the medications to find the optimal dosage. The therapeutic window is relatively large. Most patients will require less than 30 mg haloperidol, but others may require three times as much.[12] Such high-dose neuroleptization should be done only with careful monitoring of the patient.

The environmental strategies for management ensure the patient's safety

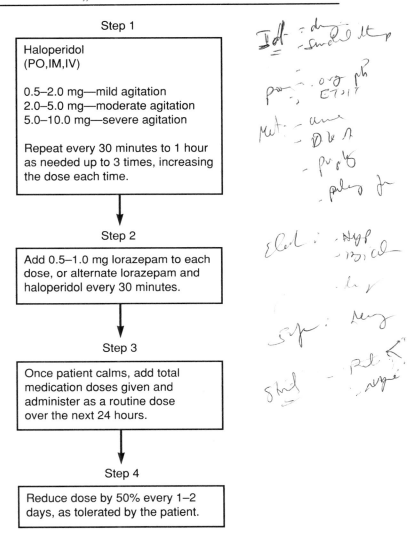

Step 1

Haloperidol
(PO,IM,IV)

0.5–2.0 mg—mild agitation
2.0–5.0 mg—moderate agitation
5.0–10.0 mg—severe agitation

Repeat every 30 minutes to 1 hour
as needed up to 3 times, increasing
the dose each time.

Step 2

Add 0.5–1.0 mg lorazepam to each
dose, or alternate lorazepam and
haloperidol every 30 minutes.

Step 3

Once patient calms, add total
medication doses given and
administer as a routine dose
over the next 24 hours.

Step 4

Reduce dose by 50% every 1–2
days, as tolerated by the patient.

Fig. 10-4 Typical dosing of neuroleptics in acute delirium or psychosis. Initial dose is determined by degree of agitation. Thiothixine has approximately one-third the potency of haloperidol; dosages should be adjusted accordingly. When administering lorazepam in Step 2, be sure to monitor respiratory drive carefully in patients with impaired pulmonary function.

and health. These strategies include constant observations and frequent reorientation. It is necessary to minimize stimulation and make the treatment setting as simple and consistent as possible. This may include assigning a consistent treatment staff to the patient on a daily basis. Other helpful maneuvers include putting day, date, time, and place remainders in the room, along with familiar objects from home (such as pillows and photographs). The activity in the ICU should also follow a regular circadian rhythm, with dimming of the patient's lights during the evening. Lights should not be completely extinguished for most sundowning patients, however. Most hospitalized patients awaken many times during the night. Organically impaired patients are often disoriented when they initially awaken, and the darkened room will heighten this disorientation.

Every ICU should be adept and knowledgeable concerning the use of physical restraints for delirious patients. Physical restraints are often the safest means of controlling acutely agitated behavior.[13] It is important to recognize that they should be viewed as temporary, and once behavioral control is gained with medications, attempts should be made to remove them. Common complications in the use of restraints include local irritation and bruising, impairment of distal circulation (especially if placed incorrectly), and reduced clearance of pulmonary secretions in some settings.[13] It is important that monitoring of circulation, vital signs, and hydration be performed frequently. If restraints are needed, it is recommended that the attending physician document their need on an ongoing basis as the only method to ensure safety in that particular clinical situation. Also, it is recommended that nursing staff maintain documentation of adequate monitoring every 15 to 30 minutes. In removing the restraints, it is useful to remove the restraints one at a time with enough time between the removals to document behavioral control. Typically, removing them at 15- to 30-minute intervals is sufficient. Such a transition allows an increase in the neuroleptics if needed.

Delirium represents at least one acute organ failure, the brain. Often, however, there is another organ failure underlying the "brain failure." The cardinal rule in caring for the delirious patient is to establish the cause of the delirium and correct it. The behavioral control is used to facilitate the diagnostic evaluation and prevent the patient from injuring themselves. Delirium represents the most urgent behavioral disorder in the ICU.

PSYCHOSIS

Psychosis is considered here because of the similarity of the clinical picture to delirium; covered here are the two general situations that occur in the ICU. The most common is a first episode of psychosis. Less commonly, a psychotic patient will present to the ICU for unrelated medical problems. Both of these situations may present problems for the ICU staff. In this section, we address the proper evaluation and treatment of the first psychotic episode. The appearance of delusional thinking and hallucinations are the most vivid symptoms of psychosis. Unlike the delirious patient, there is no clouding of consciousness. Phenomenologically, the delusional thinking represents a loss of the normal constraints of logical thinking in such a way that a pathologic thought process appears. In other words, the patient draws conclusions about his or her situation because of faulty processing of information.

Normally, a stream of thought occurs in which one thought or idea leads to the next because of some relationship. The relationship between these thoughts or ideas is constrained by logic. A delusion is a stream of thought that develops as a result of the loosening or loss of the normal logical constraints. In extreme cases, this loss of relationship is exhibited in speech patterns in which there is a so-called loosening of associations. The most extreme case of such looseness is known as "word salad." It should be apparent that thought disorders are closely related to language disorders. It should also be apparent that hallucinations are closely related to such processes as illusions and misperceptions that can occur by faulty processing in the association cortex.[8]

The evaluation of the first psychotic episode in the ICU is based on determining whether the information processing problem is the psychological result of the stress of the medical illness and its treatment, or whether it is the result of an organic illness of the brain. Take, for example, the case of a patient with word salad and delusions of alien control. How would such a patient differ from a patient with a fluent aphasia and ideomotor apraxia? In general, the distinction can often be made after a formal mental status examination and neurocortical examination. The patient with the acquired left temporal-parietal dysfunction will show "neighborhood signs," such as a visual field cut, dyscalculia, asymmetric reflexes, and cortical sensory findings.[14] Also, aphasic patients often perseverate in their speech patterns. It is necessary to evaluate the left hemisphere in patients whose psychosis is prominently displayed in their language.

Another potentially missed organic psychosis occurs in right hemispheric injuries.[4] Such patients may suffer from visual-spatial perceptual problems in such a manner that they misinterpret their environment. For example, the inability to interpret another patient's nonverbal communication is known as a receptive aprosodia.[15] This typically occurs in nondominant parietal-temporal injuries. Clinically, such patients may describe ideas of reference and paranoia. The defective function can be demonstrated by a bedside prosody examination, as described by Ross and Russ.[15]

The bedside prosody examination focuses on the spontaneous and repetitive production of affective inflections and gestures by the patient, as well as the comprehension of prosodic stimuli. The motoric aprosodias can be illustrated by asking the patient to repeat a declarative but neutrally affective statement in a happy, sad, disinterested, angry, or surprised voice. A statement that we commonly use is "I'm going to get a coke." Proper prosodic expression is more than simply raising or lowering the loudness of the voice. The spontaneous prosodic expression can be judged by asking emotionally loaded questions. Such questions should be tailored to the specific patient. For instance, to an assault victim, "Tell me about the assault." A lack of proper modulation of affective expression may appear as language devoid of emotion, or as unstable, inappropriately excessive affect. The anterior right hemisphere is associated with proper production of affective expression, and injuries in this region appear as motor aprosodias.

The posterior temporal-parietal lobe of the right hemisphere acts as an interpreter of affective expression. To evaluate the sensory prosody of the patient, the neutral declarative statement should be presented to the patient without visual cues or gestures in happy, sad, disinterested, angry, and surprised voice for the patient to interpret. Gestural prosodic interpretation may or may not be spared, and can be evaluated by producing different gestures with the hands and face for the patient to interpret. Inability to judge the affective state of others may predispose to misinterpreting the intent of others and result in paranoid thinking. Jackson noted the tendency of patients with right parietal injuries to have paranoid beliefs. It is important in new onset paranoid psychoses to establish the proper functioning of the right hemisphere. In our experience, patients with right-sided injuries are often emotionally labile and minimize their medical illness (anosagnosia). Such right hemispheric–injured patients may represent challenges for ICU staff. Both right and left hemispheric organic delusional disorders usually respond to neuroleptics.

Patients may suffer a psychotic illness as a psychological response to their medical illness. The delusions and hallucinations may be indistinguishable from organically based delusions and hallucinations. Rarely should these patients receive a diagnosis of schizophrenia. The most common diagnosis in such patients is brief reactive psychosis.[6] This is typically a short-lived psychosis following significant stress. It may be quite florid. The duration of psychosis is less than 3 months, and usually less than a few weeks. Such patients respond well to neuroleptic medications.

Rarely, other functional psychoses may appear for the first time in the ICU. This occurs with sufficient rarity that diagnosis of schizophrenia or bipolar illnesses should be made only after consultation with a psychiatrist. However, psychiatric patients also suffer medical illnesses that may result in ICU admission. In such situations, the psychiatric illness may modify the medical presentation of the patient. Some patients with schizophrenia have markedly elevated pain thresholds, such that even an acute surgical abdomen may not be suspected initially. Psychotic patients may incorporate their somatic sensations into their delusional systems. Therefore, complaints of bodily dysfunction by psychotic patients may go uninvestigated. For example, a patient may claim he or she is "possessed because the devil is in my chest squeezing my heart." This patient may be describing an acute myocardial infarction, but explains the pain as a "demonic possession." A high index of suspicion for occult medical disorders should be used in dealing with acutely decompensated psychiatric patients.

The management of psychosis in the ICU is similar to delirium. The principal aim is to both protect the patient and manage the appropriate medical care. The cornerstone of treatment is the use of neuroleptic agents. The same principles hold: titrate to effect against side effects, high-potency agents have fewer anticholinergic side effects, and lower-potency agents have more sedation. Rapidly titrating the patient during the first 24 hours with 5 to 10 mg haloperidol every hour as needed will require frequent assessment of the patient's response to the medication.[6] In general, most patients will respond at 15 to 45 mg haloperidol per day. Many, however, require higher doses. After the first 24 hours, a general idea of the medication requirements can usually be made so that routine medications can be given.

Rarely, a psychotic patient will not respond to even high-dose neuroleptics (haloperidol >100 mg/day). In such situations, the addition of lower doses of lorazepam, 1 to 2 mg, to the haloperidol is useful. Caution needs to be observed in patients who have significant respiratory problems such as chronic obstructive pulmonary disease and pneumonia.[6,16] In cases in which lorazepam is not feasible because of pulmonary problems, sedating neuroleptics such as chlorpromazine should be tried. Careful monitoring of the blood pressure is required because of adrenergic blockade side effects of chlorpromazine. Patients should be adequately hydrated when chlorpromazine is to be used.[6]

Environmental manipulations, such as those used in delirium are also useful in managing the acutely psychotic patient in the ICU. Adequate supervision of psychotic patients must be maintained until the antipsychotic agents take effect. Psychotic patients frequently have full or partial recall for the events, and may be somewhat embarrassed as the episode clears. A supportive, caring demeanor will facilitate the passing of this period.

DEPRESSION AND SUICIDE

A frequent emotional complaint in the ICU is "depression." Unfortunately, depression connotes many things. This section deals with the clinical syndromes of depression and the problem of the suicidal patient. The clinical syndromes of depression range from sadness in response to the psychosocial circumstance of the patient to melancholic depressive illness unrelated to the psychosocial circumstances of the patient. It can be conceptualized as primary or secondary.

Primary major depressive disorder, also called functional unipolar depression, is defined by a symptom profile, typical clinical course, family history, prognosis, and treatment response.[10] The most effective treatments for this condition are antidepressants.[17-19] Secondary major depressive illness shares the clinical syndrome but has identifiable etiologic factors from history, examination, or laboratory findings. Poststroke depression is one type of secondary major depressive disorder. Minor depressive illness implies a slightly less severe form of the illness.

Major depressive episodes are diagnosed based on the presence or absence of definable symptoms apparent in three areas: affective regulation, somatic concerns, and cognition.[6,10] These symptoms do not necessarily include a sad affect, although this is usually present. The affect in depressive illness typically includes a reduced reactivity of mood noticeable as a withdrawal from rewarding behaviors, which appears as social isolation, anhedonia, crying spells, and general lassitude. Cognitive complaints may include poor concentration and effort, sustained feelings of hopelessness and helplessness, and ruminations of a depressive nature; hallucinations may occur. The somatic symptoms of depressive illness may include fatigue, constipation, reduced appetite, sleep with early morning awakenings, and reduced libido. These symptoms may surface as complaints of the gastrointestinal, genitourinary, or cardiovascular systems.

The symptoms of depressive illness often interfere with the intensive care of the patient because of the negativism, and may be looked on as "personality disorders" or brushed off as "noncompliance." Untreated depressive illness has a relatively high mortality from suicide.[6]

First-line pharmacologic treatments of most primary depressive illness are the tricyclic antidepressants represented by amitriptyline, nortriptyline, imipramine, desipramine, and doxepin.[17–19] Common pharmacologic effects include blockade of the reuptake of serotonin and catecholamines, which are believed to be associated with their mechanism of action. The secondary pharmacologic effects underlie their side effects. These secondary effects include anticholinergic, antihistaminergic, and α-receptor blockade. The tricyclic antidepressants vary in the relative frequency and intensity of their secondary effects. The side effects of principal importance are orthostasis from α-blockade and anticholinergic side effects such as blurred vision, constipation, urinary retention, and a central anticholinergic delirium. Table 10-2 ranks these drugs on the basis of their relative potency in the secondary effects. Relative side effect profiles of these drugs are a consideration in drug choice. Amitriptyline is the agent associated with very high anticholinergic activity. Organically impaired patients are known to be more sensitive to the development of anticholinergic delirium. Thus, amitriptyline may prove an inappropriate choice in the ICU.

Orthostasis is an important side effect to consider in the treatment of the ICU patient. Tricyclics block peripheral α-receptors on blood vessel walls. This results in impairment of the postural reflexes. The effect noticed by the patient may range from dizziness and light-headedness to falls and fainting. The tertiary amine tricyclics such as amitriptyline, imipramine, and doxepin produce higher degrees of orthostasis.

The direct cardiac effects of the tricyclics are related to quinidine-like effects on the atrioventricular bundle and, at toxic levels, direct cardiotoxicity. Thus, introduction of tricyclic agents should be performed with caution in patients with partial or complete cardiac blocks or recent myocardial infarctions or in patients on other quinidine-like agents.[11] Fluoxetine may have a primary role in treating patients with pretreatment conduction blocks. In general, there is no reason to begin antidepressant treatment in the ICU before consultation with a psychiatrist. The onset of action usually is delayed, making their use as an emergency treatment limited. There are reports of the use of electroconvulsive therapy (ECT) in medically complicated patients such as those post–myocardial infarction.[20] In functional depression, ECT has a record of safety and efficacy but is used infrequently because of the effectiveness of tricyclics. Although safe, ECT carries the same risks as brief general anesthesia.[20] Also, the convulsion induced from ECT has physiologic effects on the cardiac system, and careful pretreatment screening is urged.[20]

A second generation of antidepressant agents has become available. Their principal advantage is not improved efficacy but improved side effect profile. The second-generation antidepressants also have a different nontricyclic-like side effects such as priapism with trazadone, seizures with maprotyline, extra-

Table 10-2. SECONDARY EFFECTS OF
TRICYCLIC ANTIDEPRESSANTS

	Reuptake		Receptor Blockade[a]		
Drug	NE	5-HT	α-1	Ach	H-1
Tertiary Amines					
Amitriptyline	+/−	+ +	+ + +	+ + +	+ + +
Imipramine	+	+	+ + +	+ +	+ +
Doxepin	+	+/−	+ +	+ +	+ + +
Secondary Amines					
Nortriptyline	+ +	+/−	+	+	+/−
Desipramine	+ + +	+/−	+ + +	+	+

Abbreviations: NE, norepinephrine; 5-HT, serotonin; α-1, α-1 adrenergic
receptors; Ach, acetylcholine receptors; H-1, histamine-1 receptors.
[a] Blockade of α-1 results in orthostatic hypotension. Blockade of Ach
results in blurred vision, urinary retention, constipation, dry mouth. Blockade of H-1 results in sedation.
(Data from Goodman and Charney[18] and Richelson.[19])

pyramidal side effects with amoxapine, and the extremely long half-life of
fluoxetine. In the treatment of the type of complicated multisystem disorders
ICU patients tend to have, these side effects may complicate overall medical/
neurological treatment. It should be emphasized that while these drugs have
a place in the treatment of depression, they are no more effective than the
classic tricyclic agents. Some of the second-generation agents are less toxic in
overdose than the tricyclic agents.[18,19] It may be reasonable for chronically
suicidal patients to be treated with these agents as first-line drugs.

THE SUICIDAL PATIENT

The suicidal patient in the ICU represents a potentially disastrous situation.
Most often, these are patients who have been hospitalized because of a recent
suicide attempt. Approximately 1 percent of the population will die as a result
of suicide.[6] Approximately two-thirds of suicide cases will have communicated
their intent to someone.[21] A large percentage will have recently seen a physician.[21] Depression and alcoholism predispose to suicide attempts. About 80
percent of completed suicides are among these diagnostic groups.[6,22] Thirty
percent to 40 percent of suicide completers have a positive blood alcohol test.[6]
Drugs such as benzodiazepines and barbiturates are commonly associated
with suicide attempts. This suggests that, in many patients, disinhibiting
drugs reduce the threshold for self-destruction.

Less well known is the high incidence of suicide in patients with physical
illnesses. These illnesses include patients with histories of traumatic brain
injuries, epilepsy, Huntington's disease, multiple sclerosis, chronic renal disease, acquired immunodeficiency syndrome (AIDS), and cancer.[6] With the
possible exceptions of epilepsy, AIDS, renal disease, and cancer, most of these
"complicated" suicidal patients arrive in the ICU for the sequelae of the suicide
method and not the underlying physical illness.

Although a psychiatric consultation for patients who have attempted suicide is strongly encouraged, the ICU physician should be familiar with the basic aspects of evaluating and managing the patient following a suicide attempt. The principal concern is whether the patient remains at risk for further attempts. The assessment of suicidal tendencies involves a complete psychiatric history and mental status examination.[6] Specifically, the physician should inquire about suicidal thoughts, feelings of hopelessness, recent losses, previous attempts, available means such as pills and firearms, and future plans. It is unsettling that only one in six clinicians asks about suicide. Most patients will discuss suicidal thoughts when asked. The physician should not fear giving a patient ideas by inquiring about suicide. The risk factors for suicide include historical, demographic, and biomedical factors. The clustering of certain psychosocial and demographic factors in suicidal patients aids the ICU physician in short-term management until formal psychiatric consultation can be obtained. Table 10-3 shows risk factors for suicide.

Any patient with a history of previous attempts should be considered at future risk. Approximately 10 percent of attempters will later complete the suicide act.[6,22] In the ICU, the attention to the suicidal patient may require around-the-clock, careful observations to avoid in-hospital suicide. Specifically, an order for suicide precautions should be entered in the physician's orders and discussed with nursing personnel. Twenty-four hour one-on-one supervision of the patient in the ICU may not be practical without extra personnel. Clear orders for one-to-one suicide precautions should be reinforced with hospital administration if necessary. Sharp objects should be removed from the patient's reach. Rarely should antidepressant therapy be started in the ICU before a psychiatric consultant is available.

After an attempt it is not unusual for patients to have sudden temporary

Table 10-3. RISK FACTORS FOR SUICIDE

Biomedical
    Chronic or debilitating medical disease
    History of traumatic brain injury

Psychological
    Previous attempts
    Alcohol or substance abuse
    History of affective illness in patient or family
    Feelings of helplessness and hopelessness
    Recent psychiatric hospitalization

Social
    White race
    Recent job loss
    Recent personal loss
    Single, widowed, or divorced
    Adolescence or old age
    Isolated living situation

Environmental
    Access to method (firearms, pills)

improvement in their mood.[6] The patient's apparent condition must be balanced with other potential risk factors for future attempts. Once stable, the suicidal patient can be transferred to the psychiatrist's care as an inpatient, or as an outpatient in some cases. The decision for outpatient treatment should be made only after the patient has been examined by the psychiatrist who will be responsible for assuming the patient's care.

SUBSTANCE-ABUSING PATIENT

Substance-abusing patients express behavioral disorders in many ways in the ICU. The most common problem behaviors in the substance-abusing patient involve intoxication, withdrawal, hostility, aggression, and depression. Depression is common in substance-abusing patients in both the intoxicated and withdrawal states.[6] We focus in this section on withdrawal and intoxication. Abused substances include alcohol, sedatives (benzodiazepines, barbiturates [i.e., "downers"]), stimulants (cocaine, amphetamines [i.e., "uppers"]), hallucinogens (PCP, LSD, mescaline), and opiates. In this section, we discuss these as they relate to ICU patients.

One of the more common behavioral problems in the ICU involving substance abuse is related to drug and alcohol withdrawal. The ICU implications of drug withdrawal involve alcohol and sedatives. Chronic use of "downers" and alcohol result in a physiologic adaptation to their presence. When they are rapidly withdrawn, a state of physiologic arousal generally appears. The behavioral disorders that appear as a result of the withdrawal range from mild anxiety to frank delirium.[23]

Withdrawal seizures may occur after withdrawal of alcohol or downers from an addict. The delirium from the withdrawal of alcohol and some sedative hypnotic agents (especially the barbiturates) is occasionally fatal. Perhaps the easiest treatment for these withdrawal seizures is prevention through a tapering dose of benzodiazepines.[6,24] Thiamine should also be given to any patient suspected of alcohol addiction. Unfortunately, a history of substance abuse is often either denied or unavailable because of the medical condition of the patient. In such situations, the treating physician may be caught off guard by the withdrawal syndrome. It is reasonable to give thiamine until a reliable history is obtainable. The objective signs of withdrawal from sedatives in the predelirious state are the result of autonomic arousal with sympathetic discharge.[6,24] The mental status components of such autonomic discharge are usually irritability and anxiety. The impact of the sympathetic arousal on the medical condition of the patient may be deleterious, resulting in volume depletion and sometimes cardiovascular collapse.

The withdrawal may also increase the patient's hostility and agitation. Although fever, tachycardia, diaphoresis, and tremor may be associated with other biomedical etiologies, their appearance should cause the ICU physician to consider the substance abuse history of the patient. Collateral history from family members, physical examination, and laboratory testing may be helpful in identifying substance abuse as a possible contributing factor in such patients. The physical examination and laboratory features of alcoholism are shown in Table 10-4.

Although similar in form, other forms of sedative withdrawal may be more prolonged and without the physical and laboratory stigmata of alcoholism.[6] In patients in whom a reliable medical and social history are unavailable, routine early testing for residual substances in the blood and urine of patients admitted to the ICU may prove invaluable in documenting the cause of later behavior problems. Once determined, appropriate withdrawal schedules can be prescribed for the patient.

Detoxification regimens for alcohol and sedatives are similar. The cross-tolerance of alcohol and the sedatives with benzodiazepines allows the physician to use tapering schedules of benzodiazepines or barbiturates.[6,24] Benzodiazepines have relatively wide therapeutic windows, with less effects on the respiratory centers than barbiturates at most therapeutic doses. This safety allows the clinician to treat withdrawal syndromes aggressively on an individualized basis.[6,24] Care should be used in treating patients with impaired pulmonary function with any sedative, including benzodiazepines.[16] The 3-hydroxy class of benzodiazepines, such as lorazepam, is useful in the ICU. Lorazepam undergoes metabolism via conjugation, without active metabolites being formed. This greatly reduces the potential for drug interactions common to the 2-keto class of benzodiazepines, such as diazepam. The half-life of lorazepam is intermediate at 10 to 20 hours.[5,6,24] This may necessitate more frequent administration during detoxification and requires greater supervision during withdrawal. Typically, 1 or 2 mg lorazepam every 1 or 2 hours as needed for the first 24 to 48 hours will safely treat most alcohol or sedative withdrawal syndromes. Usually less than 10 mg is needed, although rare patients may require more for safe detoxification. The dose can then be decreased by 10 percent to 25 percent daily over 5 to 10 days, depending on which agent was being abused. There is a wide variability in detoxification requirements, and patients should have their treatments individualized according to their response.

Table 10-4. PHYSICAL AND LABORATORY STIGMATA OF ETHANOL ABUSE

Physical Examination
  Hypertension, jaundice, increased liver span, abdominal tenderness, easy bruisability, atrial or ventricular arrhythmias, testicular atrophy, amenorrhea in women, painful and swollen muscles, spider angioma, rhinophyma, caput medusa, ascites, dementia, lability, tremor, ataxia (secondary to cerebellar degeneration), peripheral neuropathy

Laboratory
  Hematopoietic
    Megaloblastic indices, thrombocytopenia, mild anemia, decreased folate, reticulocytopenia, decreased white blood cells, hyperplastic bone marrow
  Gastrointestinal
    Increased serum glutamic oxaloacetic transaminase (SGOT), serum glutamic pyruvic transaminase (SGPT), γ-glutamyl transferase, elevated triglycerides, increased bilirubin
  Metabolic
    Hyponatremia and hypokalemia caused by solute poor fluid intake and emesis, reduced folate, reduced B-12 in setting of chronic ulcerative disease, reduced phosphates, increased uric acid, reduced magnesium, alcoholic ketoacidosis

Opiate abuse may be the result of therapeutically prescribed opiates as well as opiates purchased from the street. Opiate addiction can present problems in the ICU because of withdrawal and reduced pain threshold. The withdrawal syndrome of opiates is pharmacologically the inverse of the therapeutic effects of opiates. Opiate withdrawal is relatively easy to identify in flagrant cases. In less flagrant cases, the withdrawal is muted and appears as a reduced pain threshold with what seem to be excessive opiate analgesic requirements. The management of both situations requires tapering the opiate agents over a few days. Longer-acting opiates allow a less frequent schedule. Too short of a half-life or too infrequent dosing of the opiates results in the patient developing withdrawal symptoms repeatedly. In such situations, a positive reinforcement of the addiction can be created by rewarding the withdrawal with as-needed opiate detoxification. An alternative used by some clinicians is to withdraw the patient using clonidine at doses of 0.1 to 0.3 mg three times/day to as high as 0.7 mg three times/day.[6] Clonidine blocks the autonomic symptoms of withdrawal and may reduce opiate craving. Orthostatic hypotension often occurs with the initiation of clonidine, and appropriate care should be used. The goal of detoxification is to prevent the withdrawal syndrome.

Stimulant-abusing patients may arrive in the ICU because of a complication of the drug. Seizures are more frequent in cocaine abusers. Cardiovascular collapse and myocardial infarctions are also more frequent in stimulant abusers. Stimulant agents such as amphetamines and cocaine are associated with depressive episodes during the withdrawal phase.[6] The ICU physician can refer these patients for more definitive treatment after their medical stabilization. The principal behavioral problem for the ICU physician associated with these agents involves the intoxication state. In stimulant toxicity, a model paranoid psychosis may result.[6] The guideline given above for the treatment of psychosis should be followed. The neuroleptics are antagonistic of most of the pharmacologic effects of stimulants.[6]

A simple clinical rule is that any overdose patient should be considered a potential suicide patient. Although accidental overdose does occur, it is usually difficult to differentiate it from a suicidal overdose at first glance. As mentioned above, a recently suicidal patient may have a remarkable "flight into health" after a failed attempt. Such a patient may deny the significance of the overdose. Other risk factors for suicide, such as recent losses, notes, and depressive illness, should be considered in judging the suicidal tendencies of the substance-abusing patient.

ANXIETY IN THE INTENSIVE CARE UNIT

Anxiety is understandably common in the ICU. Its presence may be the result of a primary psychiatric disorder, a psychological response to the medical condition of the patient, or a physiologic component of an underlying medical problem or its treatment (drug-induced). In general conditions associated with sympathetic discharge or increased sympathetic responsivity are accompanied by anxiety. Table 10-5 categorizes some of the more common biomedical causes. A complete history, when available, may identify whether an anxiety disorder was present prior to the ICU admission.

Of immediate importance in some situations is the effect of the anxiety on the medical condition of the patient. Despite the potential deleterious effect of anxiety on the patient's medical condition, patients in the coronary care unit are often undertreated.[25,26] In one study, about two-thirds of the coronary care unit patients were treated with anxiolytic agents. In only 15 percent of those treated were as-needed doses administered. Even routine doses were withheld from 15 percent of patients with routine orders for anxiolytic agents.[26] Several reasons are cited for undertreatment, including fear of sedation and drug dependency and poor recognition of anxiety by treatment staff.

The benzodiazepines are the principal medication for treating anxiety in the ICU. The many different agents available allows the clinician to select between agents with high and low sedation, short or long duration of action, or oxidized or conjugated metabolic pathways. Table 10-6 illustrates the benzodiazepines and their attributes. In most situations, a relatively slow onset and low degree of sedation are preferred.

Other pharmacotherapy for anxiety often used in the ICU includes antihistamines such as phenhydramine and hydroxyzine.[24] These agents achieve their anxiolytic effect probably via mild sedation. Hydroxyzine has moderate anti-

Table 10-5. COMMON MEDICAL CAUSES
OF ANXIETY

Disease
    Cardiac
        Angina
        Congestive failure
        Arrhythmias
    Pulmonary
        Asthma, chronic obstructive pulmonary
            disease
        Hypoxia
        Embolism
    Endocrine
        Pheochromocytoma
        Thyrotoxicosis
        Hypoglycemia
    Pain
Drugs
    Bronchodilators
        Theophylline and related compounds
        Metaproteranol and related compounds
    Stimulants
    Thyroid hormones
    Decongestants
    Insulin reaction
Diet
    Caffeine
    Monosodium glutamate

Table 10-6. CHARACTERISTICS OF BENZODIAZEPINES

Benzodiazepine Class	Metabolic Pathway	Onset	Half-life (h)	Degree of Sedation
2-keto-like benzodiazepines	Hepatic oxidation with formation of active metabolites			
Diazepam		Fast	20-70	Highly
Chlorazepate		Fast	30-100	Moderately
Chlordiazepoxide		Intermediate	5-30	Moderately
Prazepam		Slow	60-70	Mildly
3-hydroxybenzodiazepines	Conjugation without active metabolites			
Lorazepam		Intermediate	10-20	Highly
Oxazepam		Slow	5-15	Mildly
Triazolobenzodiazepines	Similar to 2-keto group			
Alprazolam		Intermediate	12-15	Mildly

(Data from Wise and Cassem[5] and Andreasen and Black.[6])

cholinergic effects, such as urinary retention, that may complicate the patient's condition.[24] Hydroxyzine and phenhydramine are not recommended for first-line treatment of anxiety in most ICU patients. Also, a new agent, buspirone, which has a slow onset of action (1 to 2 weeks), is not suited for management of acute anxiety in the ICU setting.[6]

SUMMARY

The response of an individual to intensive care treatment is complicated. Loss of adaptation in the ICU results in the appearance of problem behaviors. Such behaviors are the result of the combined effects of the medical and psychological condition of the patient as well as the treatment setting. A comprehensive assessment of the patient considers the biopsychosocial elements of the patient's condition through the review of the medical record and a complete history and physical examination, including the mental status and neurocortical examination. An accurate description of the behavior and understanding of the determinants of the behavior allows the physician to categorize many of the behaviors into syndromes such as delirium, psychosis, depression, and anxiety. Specific target behaviors are identified. The effects of treatment on these target symptoms are used to judge the response. Pharmacologic and environmental manipulations in the ICU are used to maximize the patient's behavior so that the intensive medical care needed can be effectively delivered. Psychiatric consultation may facilitate the intensive care of the patient by stabilizing the behavioral condition of the patient. Such consultation should be responsive to the concerns of the ICU physician as well as the patient.

REFERENCES

1. Cassem NH, Hackett TP: The setting of intensive care. p. 353. In Hackett TP, Cassem NH (eds): Massachusetts General Hospital Handbook of General Psychiatry. 2nd Ed. PSG Publishing, Littleton, MA, 1987

2. Rabins PV, Folstein MF: Delirium and dementia: diagnostic criteria and fatality rates. Br J Psychiatry 140:149, 1982
3. Shevitz SA, Silberfard PM, Lipowski ZJ: Psychiatric consultation in a general hospital—a report of 1000 referrals. Dis Nerv Syst 37:295, 1976
4. Lishman WA: Organic Psychiatry (The Psychological Consequences of Cerebral Disorders). Blackwell Scientific Publications, Oxford, 1987
5. Wise MG, Cassem NH: Psychiatric consultation to critical care units. p. 413. In Tasman A, Goldfinger SM, Kaufman CA (eds): Review of Psychiatry. Vol. 9. American Psychiatric Press, Washington, DC, 1990
6. Andreasen NC, Black DW: Introductory Textbook of Psychiatry. American Psychiatric Press, Washington, DC, 1991
7. Folstein MF, Folstein, SE, McHugh PR: "Mini-Mental State": a practical method for grading the cognitive state of patients for the clinician. J Psychiatr Res 12:189, 1975
8. Flor-Henry P: Cerebral Basis of Psychopathology. John Wright PSG, London, 1983
9. Tesar GE, Stern TA: Evaluation and treatment of agitation in the intensive care unit. J Intensive Care Med 1:137, 1986
10. American Psychiatric Association: Diagnostic and Statistical Manual of Mental Disorders. 3rd Ed. Revised. American Psychiatric Association, Washington, DC, 1987
11. Kaplan HI, Sadock BJ: Drugs used to treat anxiety and insomnia. In: Synopsis of Psychiatry: Behavioral Sciences, Clinical Psychiatry. 5th Ed. Williams & Wilkins, Baltimore, 1988
12. Adam F: Emergency intravenous sedation of the delirious, medically ill patient. J Clin Psychiatry 49(suppl. 12):22, 1988
13. Soloff PH: Emergency management of violent patients. In Hales RE, Frances AJ (eds): Annual Review of Psychiatry. Vol. 6. American Psychiatric Press, Washington, DC, 1987
14. Geschwind N: Non-aphasic disorders of speech. Int J Neurol 4:207, 1964
15. Ross ED, Rush AJ: Diagnosis and neuroanatomical correlates of depression in brain-damaged patients, implications for a neurology of depression. Arch Gen Psychiatry 38:1344, 1981
16. Stoudemire GA, Levenson JL: Psychiatric consultation to internal medicine. p. 466. In Tasman A, Goldfinger SM, Kaufman CA (eds): Review of Psychiatry. Vol. 9. American Psychiatric Press, Washington, DC, 1990
17. Asberg M: Treatment of depression with tricyclic drugs—pharmacokinetic and pharmacodynamic aspects. Pharmakopsychiatr Neuropsychopharmakol 9:18, 1976
18. Goodman WK, Charney DS: Therapeutic applications and mechanisms of action of monamine oxidase inhibitor and heterocyclic antidepressant drugs. J Clin Psychiatry 46:6, 1985
19. Richelson E: Synaptic pharmacology of antidepressants: an update. McLean Hosp J 13:67, 1988
20. Consensus Conference: Electroconvulsive therapy. JAMA 254:2103, 1985
21. Slaby AE, Lieb J, Tancredi LR: Handbook of Psychiatric Emergencies. 2nd Ed. Medical Examination Publishing Co., New York, 1981
22. Robins E: Suicide. In Kaplan HI, Sadock BJ (eds): Comprehensive Textbook of Psychiatry. 4th Ed. Williams & Wilkins, Baltimore, 1985
23. Goodwin DW: Alcoholism and alcoholic psychosis. In Kaplan HI, Sadock BJ (eds): Comprehensive Textbook of Psychiatry. 4th Ed. Williams & Wilkins, Baltimore, 1985

24. Schatzberg AF, Cole JO: Manual of Clinical Psychopharmacology. American Psychiatric Press, Washington, DC, 1986
25. Strain JJ, Leibowitz MR, Klien DF: Anxiety and panic attacks in the medically ill. Psychiatr Clin North Am 4:333, 1981
26. Stern TA, Caplan RA, Cassem NH: Use of benzodiazepines in a coronary care unit. Psychosomatics 28:19, 1987

Index

Page numbers in italics refer to figures; those followed by t indicate tables.